AF597477

Ernst Schering Research Foundation Workshop 28
Therapeutic Angiogenesis

Springer
Berlin
Heidelberg
New York
Barcelona
Hong Kong
London
Milan
Paris
Singapore
Tokyo

Ernst Schering Research Foundation
Workshop 28

Therapeutic Angiogenesis

J.A. Dormandy, W.P. Dole, G.M. Rubanyi
Editors

With 26 Figures and 10 Tables

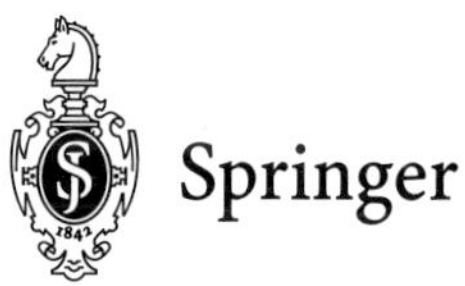

Series Editors: G. Stock and U.-F. Habenicht

ISSN 0947-6075
ISBN 3-540-65693-6 Springer-Verlag Berlin Heidelberg New York

CIP data applied for

Die Deutsche Bibliothek – CIP-Einheitsaufnahme
Schering-Forschungsgesellschaft <Berlin>: Ernst Schering Research Foundation Workshop. - Berlin; Heidelberg; New York; Barcelona; Budapest; Hong Kong; London; Milan; Paris; Santa Clara; Singapore; Tokyo: Springer.
ISSN 0947-6075
28. Therapeutic Angiogenesis. - 1999
Therapeutic Angiogenesis: from basic science to the clinic / J.A. Dormandy ... ed. - Berlin; Heidelberg; New York; Barcelona; Budapest; Hong Kong; London; Milan; Paris; Singapore; Tokyo: Springer, 1999
(Ernst Schering Research Foundation Workshop; 28)
ISBN 3-540- 65693-6

Typesetting: Data conversion by Springer-Verlag
Printing: Druckhaus Beltz, Hemsbach. Binding: J. Schäffer GmbH & Co. KG, Grünstadt
SPIN:10691227 13/3134–5 4 3 2 1 0 – Printed on acid-free paper

Preface

Over the past decade, rapid progress had been made in elucidating the cellular and molecular mechanisms of new blood vessel formation in both health and disease. Lack of sufficient angiogenesis (new capillary development) and collateral formation (remodeling of existing blood vessels) in adult tissues (e.g., heart, brain, skeletal muscle) during critical ischemia has prompted novel therapeutic strategies to stimulate/facilitate angiogenesis and collateral formation in ischemic conditions ("therapeutic angiogenesis").

Therapeutic angiogenesis describes a strategy of inducing new collateral vessels that can bypass vascular obstructions caused by atherosclerotic disease and stimulating new capillaries that can enhance tissue oxygen exchange. Naturally occurring growth factors (e.g., FGFs, VEGFs) have been identified and demonstrated to induce new blood vessel formation in the adult organism. The therapeutic application of these growth factors has been demonstrated to enhance these natural processes and have been shown in a number of animal models to increase blood flow and oxygen exchange to ischemic tissues. Therapeutic angiogenesis therefore represents a new medical principle that is anticipated to be used as an adjunct or alternative to angioplasty and/or bypass surgery. A number of strategies have been proposed and tested to deliver growth factors. One strategy is the direct administration of the growth factor protein by intramuscular, intraarterial or intravenous delivery. Gene therapy strategies using viral and non-viral vectors potentially represent a more physiologic means of delivering growth factors because they can deliver sustained, localized concentrations of the growth factor.

The Ernst Schering Foundation Workshop on Therapeutic Angiogenesis, which took place in San Francisco 18–20 October 1998, was organized to discuss the present knowledge and future directions in this important field. Leading basic scientists and clinicians reviewed and discussed several timely topics within three main themes: (1) Basic mechanisms of angiogenesis, including angiogenic growth factors and their receptors, angiopoetins and TIE receptors and extracellular matrix–endothelial cell interactions; (2) studies in experimental animal models, including collateral and capillary formation, and role of hemodynamic forces; and (3) clinical applications including various therapeutic approaches, such as protein therapy, gene therapy and transmyocardial laser therapy for treatment of myocardial ischemia, cerebral ischemia, and peripheral arterial occlusive disease.

This book contains the proceedings of the workshop. The chapters by leading experts give an excellent overview of the basic molecular aspects and clinical applications of this new emerging field. In addition to summarizing the present state of the art of therapeutic angiogenesis, this book also points out basic unanswered questions where future research is needed.

John A. Dormandy, William P. Dole, and Gabor M. Rubanyi

Table of Contents

List of Editors and Contributors

Editors

J.A. Dormandy
St. George's Hospital, Department of Vascular Surgery, Level 4,
St. James Wing, Blackshaw Road, London SW17 0QT, UK

W.P. Dole
Berlex Biosciences, 15049 San Pablo Ave., Richmond, CA 94804-0099, USA

G.M. Rubanyi
Berlex Biosciences, 15049 San Pablo Ave., Richmond, CA 94804-0099, USA

Contributors

S. F. Aranki
Brigham and Women's Hospital, Division of Cardiac Surgery,
75 Francis Street, Boston, MA 02115, USA

A. Baird
Ciblex Corporation, 11025 Roselle Street, San Diego, CA 92121, USA

M. D. Brown
Department of Sport and Exercise Science, University of Birmingham,
Birmingham B15 2TT, UK

D. A. Cheresh
Department of Immunology, The Scripps Research Institute,
10550 N. Torrey Pines Road, La Jolla, CA 92037, USA

L. H. Cohn
Brigham and Women's Hospital, Division of Cardiac Surgery,
75 Francis Street, Boston, MA 02115, USA

N. C. Cummings
Brigham and Women's Hospital, Division of Cardiac Surgery,
75 Francis Street, Boston, MA 02115, USA

E. Deindl
Max Planck Institute for Physiological and Clinical Research,
W. G. Kerckhoff-Institute, Department of Experimental Cardiology,
Benekestraße 2, D-61231 Bad Nauheim, Germany

R. L. Engler
Collateral Therapeutics Inc., 9360 Towne Centre Drive,
San Diego, CA 92121, USA

O. Hudlická
Department of Physiology, University of Birmingham Medical School,
Birmingham B15 2TT, UK

F. Mannting
Brigham and Women's Hospital, Division of Cardiac Surgery,
75 Francis Street, Boston, MA 02115, USA

K. H. Plate
Neurocenter, Freiburg University Medical School, Breisacherstrasse 64,
D-79106 Freiburg, Germany

K. S. Riddelle-Spencer
Department of Immunology, The Scripps Research Institute,
10550 N. Torrey Pines Road, La Jolla, CA 92037, USA

T. N. Sato
The University of Texas Southwestern Medical Center at Dallas,
5323 Harry Hines Blvd., Dallas, Texas 75235–8573, USA

W. Schaper
Max Planck Institute for Physiological and Clinical Research,
W. G. Kerckhoff-Institute, Department of Experimental Cardiology,
Benekestraße 2, D-61231 Bad Nauheim, Germany

S. P. Sears
Brigham and Women's Hospital, Division of Cardiac Surgery,
75 Francis Street, Boston, MA 02115, USA

S. K. Shernan
Brigham and Women's Hospital, Division of Cardiac Surgery,
75 Francis Street, Boston, MA 02115, USA

M. Simons
Angiogenesis Research Center, Harvard Medical School,
Beth Israel Deaconess Medical Center, 330 Brookline Ave.,
Boston, MA 02215, USA

S. Ylä-Herttuala
A. I. Virtanen Institute and Department of Medicine, University of Kuopio,
P.O. Box 1627, FIN-70211 Kuopio, Finland

1 Angiogenesis, Fibroblast Growth Factors, and Their Receptors

A. Baird

1.1 Overview

The key determinants defining the earliest events in angiogenesis, vasculogenesis, and the molecular differences that distinguish arteries from veins are now better understood than at any time to date. The adult vasculature consists of large arteries that progressively branch into smaller and smaller vessels terminating into precapillary arterioles that eventually give rise to capillaries. These relatively simple structures consist of essentially one cell type, the endothelial cell, although often there are associated pericytes. Feeding into postcapillary venules, the complete network consists of progressively larger venous structures.

The earliest stage of vascular development, termed vasculogenesis, is characterized by the de novo formation of blood vessels. Here, the role played by the vascular endothelial cell growth factor (VEGF) has been clearly established by knockout of the gene. In affected animals, no vasculature is formed and embryonic lethality is observed. In contrast, when the angiopoietin gene is knocked out, a vasculature appears; but lethality ensues because it fails to develop. Similar studies with FGF2 fail to reveal any embryonic effects, although the adult animals have altered vascular tone. Hence, VEGF is viewed as a major, perhaps the most critical, angiogenic factor. Although the FGFs remain the most potent angiogenic factors described so far (see below), if they play a role, it is not during development. In this review, the FGF family is reviewed and their role in angiogenesis and angiogenesis-dependent events evaluated.

Fibroblast growth factors (FGFs) represent a large family of polypeptides that are potent regulators of cell growth and differentiation (Galzie et al. 1997; Coulier et al. 1997; Burgess and Marciag 1989). While they play a major role in normal embryonic development, and tissue repair and regeneration, they have also been implicated in numerous pathologies, including the development and progression of several malignancies. FGFs act on cells that are primarily of mesodermal origin, but have broader effects on cells derived from ectoderm and endoderm. Depending on the target cell, the conditions of cell culture, and the presence or absence of other trophic agents, FGFs alter migration, morphology, differentiation, and proliferation (Baird and Klagsbrun 1991a). While first discovered for their effect on fibroblasts (hence their name), their physiological roles and behavior are considerably more extensive than their name implies. In fact, some members of the FGF family are not even mitogens for fibroblasts at all and would be better represented as epithelial growth factors.

To date, the family of FGFs consists of 17 genes encoding proteins that have 30–80% structural homology at the amino acid level (Fig. 1). More may be identified as the human genome becomes fully characterized. The interleukins 1α and -β, which have 20% homology with FGF1 and FGF2, are not usually considered members of the FGF family, even though they have a number of features in common with the FGFs, including a similar tertiary structure. While the members of the FGF family are designated FGF1 through FGF17, the names of acidic FGF (FGF1), basic FGF (FGF2), and KGF (keratinocyte growth factor, FGF7) are also commonly used in the literature. Other names for FGFs such as int2 (FGF3), hst1/ksFGF/kFGF (FGF4), hst2 (FGF6), androgen-induced growth factor (FGF8), and glial activating factor (FGF8)

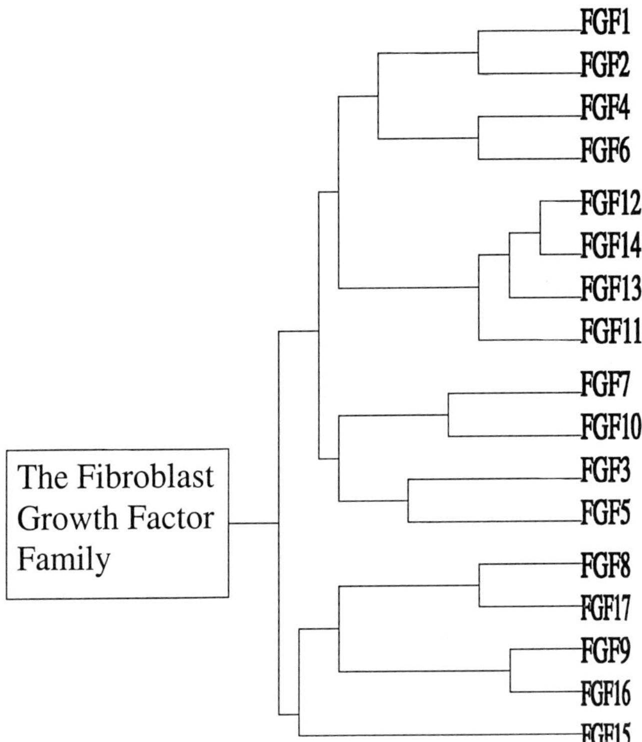

Fig. 1. Phylogenic tree outlining the structural similarities between FGFs. The length of all lines is proportional to the structural homology between FGF family members. Presumably derived from a common ancestral gene, the mammalian FGF family has evolved to include over 18 different genes (From Hoshikawa et al. 1998)

are used only rarely as the nomenclature describing the FGF family becomes standardized (Coulier et al. 1997; Baird and Klagsbrun 1991b).

There are four high affinity receptors for FGFs encoded by distinct genes. Called FGFR1, FGFR2, FGFR3, and FGFR4 respectively, the genes encode a multitude of structural variants that result from alternative splicing of their mRNAs. As a result, the specificity of ligand binding can be drastically modified by generating different spliced forms. The best example is FGF7, also known as KGF, which does not crossreact with any FGFR except a variant of FGFR2. Accordingly, it is very specific (Finch et al. 1989; Miki et al. 1991).

The basic structure is the same for all FGFRs; they belong to the immunoglobulin (Ig)-like family of tyrosine kinases. All possess three Ig-like domains that can be processed to isoforms that contain two Ig-like domains connected to an intracellular tyrosine kinase domain activated by ligand binding. In some instances, genetic mutations in the transmembrane domain result in constitutive activation and, in humans, various forms of dwarfism (Shiang et al. 1994; Bonaventure et al. 1996).

The FGF ligand-FGF receptor interaction is further complicated by the role of proteoglycans in FGF action. Specifically, FGFs have an unusually high affinity for heparan sulfates, which translates into the ability to interact with glycosaminoglycans, like heparin. This binding causes conformational changes in the FGFs that result in altered receptor binding, and protects the ligand from proteolysis and acid denaturation (Prestrelski et al. 1992; Gospodarowicz and Cheng 1986). Most importantly, this interaction appears necessary for significant ligand-receptor binding. Because extracellular FGF binds to heparan sulfate proteoglycans in the matrix and at the cell surface, this binding is thought to protect the FGFs and serve as a reservoir of FGFs available after trauma, injury, or any pathophysiological event that might require a rapid mobilization of FGF activity (like angiogenesis). In this model, the release of matrix-degrading enzymes during embryonic development, tissue injury, and after cell transformation to the cancer phenotype can serve to generate free, biologically active FGFs from these sites of sequestration (Vlodavsky et al. 1991; Bashkin et al. 1989). As some of the most powerful mitogens known, the FGFs appear to play key roles in significant human diseases, like cancer.

1.2 The FGF Family of Growth Factors

The number of ligands listed in the FGF family is increasing and, as sequencing of the human genome has accelerated, the discovery of new, structurally related proteins is likely to continue. They are thought to derive from a common ancestral gene (Fig. 1) and they all share a common structure of three exons separated by two short introns. They

Table 1. Chromosome location of FGFs and their receptors

Protein	Alternate names	Chromosome (human)	Locus	Reference
FGF1	Acidic FGF	5	q31–33	Jaye et al. 1986
FGF2	Basic FGF	4	q25–27	Mergia et al. 1986
FGF3	Int-2	11	q13	Nguyen et al. 1988
FGF4	ksFGF/K-FGF/hst-1	11	q13	Nguyen et al. 1988
FGF5	hst-2	4	q21	Dionne et al. 1990
FGF6	——	12	p13	De Lapeyriere et al. 1990
FGF7	KGF	15	q15–21	Mattei et al. 1995
FGF8	AIGF	10	q24–26	White et al. 1995
FGF9	GDGF	13	q11–12	Mattei et al. 1995
FGF10	——	5	p13–12	Emoto et al. 1997
FGF11	FHF-3	17	q21	Verdier et al. 1997
FGF12	FHF-1	3	q28	Verdier et al. 1997
FGF13	FHF-2	X	q26	Lovec et al. 1997
FGF14	FHF-4	13	q34	Smallwood et al. 1996
FGF15	——	——	——	——
FGF16	——	——	——	——
FGF17	——	——	——	——
FGFR1	flt2, flg	8	p11.2–11.1	Wood et al. 1995
FGFR2	KGFR, bek	10	q26	Dionne et al. 1992
FGFR3	——	4	p16.3	Keegan et al. 1993
FGFR4	——	5	q35.1-qter	Warrington et al. 1992

are located on different chromosomes (Table 1) and appear highly regulated, presumably to control malignancy. In normal, adult tissues, the predominant FGF gene products found are FGF1 and FGF2. While the functional roles played by all FGFs are currently under active investigation, significantly less is known about the more recently characterized molecules.

1.2.1 FGF1 and FGF2

Acidic and basic FGFs (now called FGF1 and FGF2, respectively) are the prototypic members of the FGF family. Named for their different isoelectric points when first detected in, and purified from, tissue extracts, they have similar molecular weights and more than 50% structural homology. Both have been isolated from numerous tissues and are the subject of extensive reviews (Galzie et al. 1997; Coulier et al. 1997; Burgess and Maciag 1989; Baird and Klagsbrun 1991a).

The gene for FGF1 is located on chromosome 5 and yields several mRNAs that differ in their 5' untranslated regions but not in their coding sequences (Renaud et al. 1996). Therefore, it is likely that different elements control mRNA translation in different tissues. In contrast, the mRNA encoding human FGF2 derives from a gene on chromosome 4 and encodes four proteins that all contain an identical core of the FGF2 protein sequence (Abraham et al. 1986; Florkiewicz and Sommer 1989). The three amino terminally extended forms of FGF2 extend the 18 kDa molecule of 155 amino acids to proteins of 21, 22, and 25 kDa. These isoforms translocate to the nucleus, where they are thought to play a role in controlling transcription. The lowest molecular weight FGF2 is cytoplasmic and, while it can be released from cells, it appears to follow an unconventional release pathway (Florkiewicz et al. 1995; Mignatti and Rifkin 1991). Unlike many of the other FGFs and all classically secreted proteins, both FGF1 and FGF2 lack a classical leader sequence and do not exit the cell through the endoplasmic reticulum (ER) Golgi apparatus complex.

Both FGF1 and FGF2 stimulate the proliferation of mesodermal cells and many cells of neuroectodermal, ectodermal, and endodermal origin. They are also characterized by the wide array of activities that they can stimulate on different cell types (Baird 1993). While they are perhaps best known as powerful angiogenic factors (because of their effects on endothelial cells), they also modulate differentiated function, delay senescence, inhibit apopotosis, and are chemotactic, depending on the in vitro cell system used, the conditions of cell culture, and the target cell evaluated. In vivo, these FGFs are active in angiogenesis, nerve regeneration, cartilage repair, and wound healing, and are thought to fulfill normal functions in tissue repair and homeostasis. Observations that an inappropriate expression of FGFs can result in tumor growth and development (see below) suggest that they also participate in the production of a large variety of pathogenic conditions that are angiogenesis-dependent or result in cell proliferation.

1.2.2 FGF3

Following the structural characterization of FGF1 and FGF2, various databases could be evaluated for the presence of homologous proteins.

The first of these FGFs so identified was int2 (Yoshida et al. 1987). Int2 (now called FGF3) was first recognized as a cellular gene activated after integration of the mouse mammary tumor virus into the mouse genome. The gene is located on chromosome 11 (Table 1) and encodes a protein of 240 amino acids that has about 40% homology to FGFs1 and -2. An extension at the amino terminus includes a classical leader sequence that allows it to be secreted through the ER Golgi but, interestingly, alternative forms of its mRNA encode an FGF3 with no leader sequence. These isoforms remain inside the cell where they are translocated to the nucleus to play a role in regulating gene transcription. The elements that decide which form of FGF3 is to be produced have not been defined. The secreted form of FGF3 derives from a classical AUG codon, while the cellular form is derived when this AUG is overridden by the use of an alternative start site at a CUG codon.

The regulation of FGF3 transcription appears to be coordinated by three distinct promoters and two alternative polyadenylation sites. The gene generates six different RNA species, all with the same coding capacity, but FGF3 has two, alternative upstream initiation codons in which a CUG is the major start site for FGF3. A downstream AUG codon initiates translation of the shorter 30.5 kDa protein. A number of replacement and deletion mutations have shown that the amino terminal extension is crucial for nuclear import, although the nuclear targeting signals are located elsewhere in the protein. The decision whether to enter the secretory pathway or the nucleus appears to depend on a balance of competing signals involving the amino terminus, a signal peptide, and the nuclear localization sequence. The relative position of the signaling motifs is also an important factor in establishing the proportion of FGF3 destined for the different intracellular compartments. Unfortunately, the physiological activities of FGF3 are ill-defined, but it is thought to play a role in embryonic development (Wilkinson et al. 1988, 1989).

1.2.3 FGF4

When the genomic fragments of the human tumor-derived oncogene hst1 were sequenced, and the oncogene derived from a Kaposi's sarcoma cell line was characterized, they were found to encode the same

206 amino acid protein with 40% homology to FGF1, FGF2, and FGF3. First called K-FGF or hst1, it is now commonly known as FGF4 (Yoshida et al. 1987; Delli Bovi et al. 1987) and is located on human chromosome 11 in close proximity to FGF3 (Table 1). The amino terminus of FGF4 is extended when compared to FGF1 and FGF2, and the extension includes a leader sequence for secretion through the ER Golgi. The mature protein is glycosylated, secreted, and transforming. It occurs with high frequency in some tumors, such as in the stomach, and is found during normal embryonic development. Like FGF1 and FGF2, it is a highly angiogenic molecule. Unlike the prototypic FGFs, it is rare in adult tissues but is thought to play a role in limb development (Niswander et al. 1994) and somite patterning (Grass et al. 1996).

1.2.4 FGF5

The fifth member of the FGF family was identified from a cDNA library prepared from bladder cancer that was screened for transforming oncogenes (Zhan et al. 1988). The encoded protein was found to have 40% homology to FGF1 and FGF2, hence making it FGF5. This 267 amino acid protein has a leader sequence and, as such, is secreted from cells through the ER Golgi , as are FGF3 and -4. For this reason, it is a transforming molecule that is found in many human tumor cell lines. It is a highly angiogenic protein normally found in embryonic development, in the brain, muscles, and the heart. However, the amount of this protein found in adult tissues is low when compared to FGF1 and FGF2, although it is detectable.

The gene encoding human FGF5 has alternative polyadenylation sites from which two main RNA species of 1.6 and 1.4 kb are transcribed (Zhan et al. 1988). The regulatory elements of transcription have yet to be identified, but there is evidence for translational control of FGF5 expression. The FGF5 mRNA contains a short, out-of-frame open reading frame (ORF) upstream of the ORF coding for the growth factor. Deletion of the upstream ORF enhances FGF5 translation and transforming ability, supporting the observation that FGF5 is mitogenic and overexpressed in some human cancers.

1.2.6 FGF6

The sixth FGF was first detected as hst2 and as a cDNA that cross-hybridized with probes encoding FGF4 (Iida et al. 1992; Marics et al. 1989). As a result, an FGF was sequenced that has 70% homology with FGF4 and about 30% homology with FGF1 and -2. While relatively little is known regarding the activities of FGF6 in vivo, it is known to be angiogenic, transforming when expressed in cells, and normally found during embryonic development, where it presumably mediates many activities first ascribed to FGF1 and FGF2. Because FGF6 exhibits a restricted expression profile that is dominant in the myogenic lineage (Han and Martin 1993), important functions in wound healing and tissue regeneration have been suggested (Floss et al. 1997). Like the FGFs with oncogenic potential, FGF6 has a leader sequence at its amino terminus that enables ER Golgi-dependant secretion.

1.2.7 FGF7

One of the most-studied FGFs, FGF7 is unlike the other FGF mitogens in that it shows significant specificity for epithelial cells (Finch et al. 1989). First identified as keratinocyte growth factor (KGF), it has no effect on many cells considered the usual targets for FGFs (i.e., endothelial cells). Because of its cell- and receptor (FGFR2) specificity, KGF/FGF7 has no angiogenic activity. Its gene encodes a protein with an amino terminus that has a leader sequence for secretion and a 22 kDa protein with 35% homology to the other FGFs. Its mRNA is found in a number of stromal fibroblast cell lines derived from embryonic and adult tissues, but is absent from epithelial cells. Of all the FGFs, FGF7 has the clearest paracrine function, as it is always produced in stromal cells but acts only on target epithelial cells (Aaronson et al. 1991). If it is produced in cells that express the receptor (see below), it is transforming. The specific isoform of FGF receptor that binds FGF7, however, is highly restricted in distribution and found almost exclusively on epithelial cells. Aberrant expression leads to proliferative disease.

There is a canonical TATA box 30 nucleotides upstream of its transcription initiation site. Physiological FGF7 transcription is regulated developmentally by an enhancer element located in the 3’ untranslated region of exon 3. This enhancer contains a series of consensus binding sites for a number of known transcription factors, including SP1 and AP1. Although it is probable that the specific *trans* factors controlling expression of the gene for FGF7 belong to the family of octamer-binding proteins (some known to be developmentally regulated), there is no evidence to date for post-transcriptional or post-translational control of FGF7 expression.

1.2.8 FGF8

When the activity induced by androgen-treated Shionogi carcinoma cells was isolated and characterized, the molecule was found to have 30–40% homology with other members of the FGF family. It was called FGF8 (Gemel et al. 1996; Tanaka et al. 1992). The gene, located on human chromosome 10 (Table 1), encodes a protein with a leader peptide and for this reason the molecule is found in conditioned media of FGF8-producing cells. While relatively little is known about FGF8, it is found during embryonic development and appears to play a key role in pattern development. Because of the spatiotemporal pattern of gene expression and the distribution of FGF8 protein immunoreactivity during development, it is likely that FGF8 is the true natural growth factor responsible for some activities first ascribed to FGF1 and FGF2 during embryonic development. Its distribution and expression pattern suggest a role in outgrowth and patterning of limb development (Vogel et al. 1996; White et al. 1995).

1.2.9 FGF9

First identified in cell culture supernatants as a glial activating factor (Miyamoto et al. 1993), FGF9 has 30% homology with the other FGFs and, with the exception that it stimulates proliferation and activation of glial cells and other cells expressing FGF receptors, relatively little is known regarding its physiological function. Because FGF9 has relatively higher specificity for FGFR3 than the other FGFs (Hecht et al. 1995), it is likely to be the ligand responsible for the numerous skeletal disorders associated with the FGF axis. Its ability to transform cells when overexpressed (Matsumoto-Yoshitomi et al. 1997) supports the hypothesis that it may also be involved in the development of human malignancies.

1.2.10 FGF10

Emoto et al. (1997) isolated a cDNA encoding a novel member of the FGF family that is most related to FGF7 (KGF). Like FGF7, FGF10 is mitogenic for keratinizing epidermal cells and essentially inactive on fibroblasts. Located on chromosome 5p13-p12, little is known regarding its activities, but recent studies have established that, like FGF7, it is involved in wound healing (Tagashira et al. 1997) and embryonic development (Beer et al. 1997). FGF10 appears to be differentially regulated and, like other FGFs, spacially restricted in its expression (Hattori et al. 1997).

1.2.11 FGF11, -12, -13, and -14

Using degenerate PCR and random DNA sequencing, Smallwood et al. (1996) identified four additional members of the FGF family, referred to as fibroblast growth factor homologous factors (FHFs). The genes encode proteins that are 30% homologous to other FGFs, although they have as much as 70% homology between themselves. Their physiological functions are not known but they all contain nuclear localization sequences and lack signal peptides. They are expressed primarily in the nervous system, although a comprehensive analysis of protein distribution and gene expression has not been reported. It is assumed that they play a role in nervous system development and function, but their presence in heart and connective tissues implies a broader, possibly intracellular function (Hartung et al. 1997).

1.2.12 FGF15

When McWhirter et al. (1997) characterized the downstream targets of the homeodomain oncoprotein E2A-Pbx1, they identified a new member of the FGF family, FGF15. When the deduced sequence of FGF15 was compared to other FGF family members, 30% homology was observed, the greatest similarity being between FGF15 and FGF7 and the least between FGF15 and FGF8. FGF15 also shares a common gene structure with other FGFs: three exons separated by two introns located at exactly the same homologous sequence. Like many of the other FGFs, but unlike FGF1, FGF2, and the FHFs, FGF15 has a signal sequence for targeting to the ER Golgi for secretion. Remarkably, FGF15 is not transforming under these circumstances, suggesting that it does not mediate the effects of E2A-Pbx1 on 3T3 cells. In view of its similarity to FGF7 and the fact that 3T3 cells have no receptor that crossreacts with FGF7, the findings also suggest that 3T3 cells do not possess a receptor for FGF15, but perhaps the same FGFone as for FGF7, FGFR2.

Although little is known regarding the physiological functions of FGF15, E2A-Pbx1 binds directly to a site proximal to its promoter, and the Pbx1 homeodomain is required for induction. The expression pattern of FGF15 suggests that it may play a specialized role in the nervous system. It first appears in the neuroectoderm soon after neurulation and remains restricted throughout development but never overlaps with the two other, similarly restricted FGFs, FGF3 and -8.

1.2.13 FGF16

A cDNA encoding a novel member (207 amino acids) of the FGF family from the rat heart was identified by homology-based PCR (Miyake et al. 1998). FGF16 is most similar (73% amino acid identity) to FGF9 and, like FGF9, lacks a typical signal sequence; yet it is efficiently secreted by Sf9 insect cells infected with recombinant baculoviruses containing the FGF16 cDNA. FGF16 mRNA is predominantly expressed among adult tissues in the rat heart. In rat embryos, FGF16 mRNA is predominantly expressed in the brown adipose tissue, but expression decreases greatly after birth. Whether FGF16 might be a novel secreted FGF that plays a role in development of the brown adipose tissue is unknown.

1.2.14 FGF17

A cDNA encoding a novel member (216 amino acids) of the FGF family was identified in rat embryos by Ito's laboratory soon after their characterization of FGF16 (Hoshikawa et al. 1998). Among FGF family members, FGF17 is most similar (53.7% amino acid identity) to FGF8. FGF17 has a typical signal sequence at its amino terminus. FGF17 mRNA of approximately 2.1 kb is detected in rat embryos at E14.5, but not at E10.5 or E19.5. It is found to be preferentially expressed in the neuroepithelia of the isthmus and septum of the rat embryonic brain at E14. Whether FGF17 might be a novel secreted molecule involved in the induction and patterning of the embryonic brain is unknown.

1.3 High Affinity FGF Receptors

The FGF receptor family is one of several subclasses of tyrosine kinase receptors that includes four members encoded by distinct genes: FGFR1 (sometimes called flg or fms-like), FGFR2 (sometimes called bek or bacterial expressed kinase), FGFR3 and FGFR4 (Galzie et al. 1997).

The FGFRs contain a single membrane spanning domain, an extracellular domain, and an intracellular domain that has tyrosine kinase activity and is itself phosphorylated. The extracellular domain is characterized by three Ig-like domains, although each receptor gene can produce mRNA encoding smaller receptors with two or even only one Ig domain.

The complexity of the receptor family is increased by a differential RNA splicing dictated by the exon structures of each gene. For example, no fewer than six different classes of FGFR1s can be produced from the gene encoding this receptor. They either have no secretory signal sequence, deletion of the first Ig loop, alternative splicing into the third Ig loop, deletions prior to the third Ig loop, or truncation of the transmembrane domain to generate a soluble FGFR1. Together with the isoforms generated by the genes for FGFR2 and FGFR3, there are over 100 different combinations possible at the cell surface.

The various isoforms of FGF receptors have different binding affinities for different FGF ligands (Ornitz and Leder 1992; Ornitz et al. 1996;

Blunt et al. 1997). Even the secreted form of FGFR1 is capable of binding FGF2, but not FGF1. Because the third Ig loop appears to confer selectivity, FGF1, FGF2, or sometimes both, will interact with FGFR1. When FGFR2 is spliced in the third Ig loop, it generates a receptor that recognizes FGF7 and FGF1, but not FGF2–6 and FGF8–9. Similarly, FGF8 and FGF9 appear to have increased selectivity for FGFR3 (Chellaiah et al. 1994). The isoforms of truncated receptors can act either as binding proteins secreted in the absence of a transmembrane domain or as dominant negative receptors when trapped at the cell surface. Data is only beginning to surface that suggests that different FGFRs might have different signaling roles. FGFR1 is often associated, and the other receptors somewhat less so, with malignancies and transformation. In any event, because signaling requires receptor dimerization, the complexity of the FGFR response is compounded by the possibility that heterogeneous dimers have different ligand specificity and altered intracellular substrates for tyrosine phosphorylation than the homodimers.

1.4 Low Affinity Receptors

If the number of FGF ligands and high affinity receptor isoforms were not enough to create significant complexity, the low affinity receptors interacting with FGFs at the cell surface add yet more. Firstly, low affinity receptors bind FGFs with relative high affinity (1–20 nM) so that they are thought to play an important role in controlling their activities (Galzie et al. 1997). FGF binding to all heparan sulfate proteoglycans (HSPGs) can be considered low only when they are compared to FGF high affinity receptors (Kd 1–10 pM). These HSPGs can be at the cell surface, in the extracellular matrix, or dissolved in biological fluids. They consist of a core protein to which a variable number of glycosaminoglycan chains are linked. Depending on the core protein, HSPGs can be syndecans, glypicans, perlecans, or betaglycans, each with its own spectrum of FGF binding, localization in tissues, developmental expression pattern, and ability to control FGF activity. Located in biological fluids, on the cell surface, and extracellular matrix, they can sequester FGFs to either block interactions with their receptors, deliver FGFs to their high affinity receptors to form a receptor complex, or simply stabilize the mitogens so that they are protease resistant and acid stable in a wound healing milieu.

The sequestering function of HSPGs is probably best described for FGF2. Analyses of cells in culture, tissue sections of developing and adult tissues, and biochemical studies have all pointed to the localization of FGF2 in basement membranes, where it is bound to HSPGs (Vlodavsky et al. 1987). Here, there are many binding sites that serve to restrict the diffusion of FGF2 to other tissues and cellular compartments. The HSPG interaction may also have a regulatory role, since the depot of mitogen allows slow and gradual release to the high affinity receptor. Accordingly, degradation of basement membranes during wound healing and tissue repair, embryonic development, tumor growth, and metastasis provokes release of FGFs and increases their availability to cells expressing high affinity receptors (Vlodavsky et al. 1991; Bashkin et al. 1989). Because the binding of FGFs to HSPGs is sequence-specific, their interaction is also independently controlled from other heparin-binding proteins, such as hepatocyte growth factor, antithrombin, and TGFβs, to name a few.

In addition to the storage and sequestration functions of HSPGs in the control of FGF activities, there is compelling evidence that the HSPGs, with the high affinity receptor, play a role in the signal transduction cascade (Klagsbrun and Baird 1991). When cells are chemically, enzymatically, or genetically stripped of their cell surface HSPGs, they are no longer responsive to FGFs unless the heparin GAG is also added to the cells. Accordingly, the formation of a heteromultimeric receptor complex possibly consisting of several high and low affinity receptors and ligands appears to be responsible for binding, internalization, and cell responsiveness to FGFs. Based on the need for dimerization of high affinity receptors in order to elicit a mitogenic response, the signaling complex most likely includes at least two high affinity receptors, two HSPGs, and two ligands. Moreover, with the possibility of heterodimerization, specificity and responsiveness could be altered when FGFR1 dimerizes with another FGFR, for example FGFR3, at the cell surface. The generation of numerous molecular isoforms for each gene product underscores the complexity of the FGF-FGFR axis.

1.5 FGFs in Angiogenesis

Although there are now 17 FGFs described in the literature, the bulk of all work has been performed with FGF1 and -2. Yet, both these mitogens are devoid of a signal peptide, are not secreted from cells through the ER Golgi, and have no transforming activity when overexpressed in cells. But they are nearly ubiquitous in distribution, associated with numerous cell types, powerful mitogens for tumor cells, and the most potent angiogenic factors by far. FGF2 has been demonstrated in a number of neoplastic cells, both in culture and in tissues. This is of significant interest because of its intrinsic angiogenic activity and its ability to stimulate, in what is presumed to be an autocrine fashion, the tumor cells themselves. With its wide distribution in normal cells and its detection in adrenal pheochromocytomas, renal carcinoma, bladder carcinoma, brain tumors and astrocytomas, hepatocytomas, breast and prostate cancer, and carcinoma of the digestive tract and melanoma, it must be highly regulated, presumably at the time of its release from cells. The transforming FGFs that have signal peptides and are released from cells through the ER Golgi may also be significant pathogenic agents. As a very specific growth factor for melanocytes, FGF2 mRNA appears during transformation to the malignant phenotype because the transformed cells are no longer dependent on the presence of exogenous growth factor (Halabran et al. 1988).

In contrast, some of the other FGFs were characterized on the basis of their ability to transform cells in culture. They are most often observed during embryonic development and fetal differentiation, but are also detected in a very restricted fashion in selected adult tissues. To date, there is little clear evidence to fully link any one of these FGFs with any particular form of cancer, but examples have been reported. FGF3 is activated by proviral insertion in some viral-induced mammary tumors (Peters et al. 1989) and accelerates mammary carcinogenesis (Clausse et al. 1993). It is also amplified in women with epithelial ovarian cancer (Rosen et al. 1993). It is constitutively expressed in tumorigenic but not in nontumorigenic colon carcinoma cells (Galdemard et al. 1995), and aberrant expression has been described in ovarian, breast, and endometrial tumors (Schmitt et al. 1996). While this evidence supports a circumstantial link between FGFs and transformation, antibody studies implicate a direct FGF action in the process of carcinogenesis (Talarico et al. 1990). Moreover, molecular studies have established that cell transformation is dependent on the release of FGFs from cells so that a full autocrine circuit is complete.

1.6 Conclusions

Although highly complex, the FGF family represents a group of structurally related growth factors that are among the most powerful mitogens known. They affect the function of many cell types and modulate numerous basic mechanisms of cell homeostasis. Their participation in angiogenesis can be direct, as transforming agents produced by cancer cells. Alternatively, they have profound effects on tumor growth through their control of stromal cell function and endothelial cells. Once fully understood, elucidation of the molecular mechanisms that regulate expression of these genes, and hence their biological activities, will allow the creation of innovative new strategies for the control and prevention of cancer.

References

Aaronson SA, Bottaro DP, Miki T et al (1991) Keratinocyte growth factor: a fibroblast growth factor family member with unusual target cell specificity. Ann NY Acad Sci 638:62–77

Abraham JA, Mergia A, Whang JL et al (1986) Nucleotide sequence of a bovine clone encoding the angiogenic protein, basic fibroblast growth factor. Science 233:545–548

Baird A (1993) Fibroblast growth factors: what's in a name? Endocrinology 132:487–488

Baird A, Klagsbrun M (1991a) The fibroblast growth factor family. Cancer Cells 3:239–243

Baird A, Klagsbrun M (1991b) The fibroblast growth factor family: an overview. Ann NY Acad Sci 638:xi–xii

Bashkin P, Doctrow S, Klagsbrun M, Svahn CM, Folkman J, Vlodavsky I (1989) Basic fibroblast growth factor binds to subendothelial extracellular matrix and is released by heparitinase and heparin-like molecules. Biochemistry 28:1737–1743

Beer HD, Florence C, Dammeier J, McGuire L, Werner S, Duan DR (1997) Mouse fibroblast growth factor 10: cDNA cloning, protein characterization, and regulation of mRNA expression. Oncogene 15:2211–2218
Blunt AG, Lawshé A, Cunningham ML, Seto ML, Ornitz DM, MacArthur CA (1997) Overlapping expression and redundant activation of mesenchymal fibroblast growth factor (FGF) receptors by alternatively spliced FGF8 ligands. J Biol Chem 272:3733–3738
Bonaventure J, Rousseau F, Legeai-Mallet L, Le Merrer M, Munnich A,Maroteaux P (1996) Common mutations in the fibroblast growth factor receptor 3 (FGFR 3) gene account for achondroplasia, hypochondroplasia, and thanatophoric dwarfism. Am J Med Genet 63:148–154
Burgess WH, Maciag T (1989) The heparin-binding (fibroblast) growth factor family of proteins. Annu Rev Biochem 58:575–606
Chellaiah AT, McEwen DG, Werner S, Xu J, Ornitz DM (1994) Fibroblast growth factor receptor (FGFR) 3. Alternative splicing in immunoglobulin-like domain III creates a receptor highly specific for acidic FGF/FGF1. J Biol Chem 269:11620–11627
Clausse N, Baines D, Moore R, Brookes S, Dickson C,Peters G (1993) Activation of both Wnt-1 and FGF3 by insertion of mouse mammary tumor virus downstream in the reverse orientation: a reappraisal of the enhancer insertion model. Virology 194:157–165
Coulier F, Pontarotti P, Roubin R, Hartung H, Goldfarb M, Birnbaum D (1997) Of worms and men: an evolutionary perspective on the fibroblast growth factor (FGF) and FGF receptor families. J Mol Evol 44:43–56
De Lapeyriere O, Rosnet O, Benharroch D et al (1990) Structure, chromosome mapping and expression of the murine FGF6 gene. Oncogene 5:823–832
Delli Bovi P, Curatola AM, Kern FG, Greco A, Ittman M, Basilico C (1987) An oncogene isolated by transfection of Kaposi's sarcoma DNA encodes a growth factor that is a member of the FGF family. Cell 50:729–737
Dionne CA, Kaplan R, Seuánez H, O'Brien SJ, Jaye M (1990) Chromosome assignment by polymerase chain reaction techniques: assignment of the oncogene FGF5 to human chromosome 4. Biotechniques 8:190–194
Dionne CA, Modi WS, Crumley G, O'Brien SJ, Schlessinger J, Jaye M (1992) BEK, a receptor for multiple members of the fibroblast growth factor (FGF) family, maps to human chromosome 10q25.3–q26. Cytogenet Cell Genet 60:34–36
Emoto H, Tagashira S, Mattei MG et al (1997) Structure and expression of human fibroblast growth factor-10. J Biol Chem 272:23191–23194
Finch PW, Rubin JS, Miki T, Ron D,Aaronson SA (1989) Human KGF is FGF-related with properties of a paracrine effector of epithelial cell growth. Science 245:752–755

Florkiewicz RZ, Sommer A (1989) Human basic fibroblast growth factor gene encodes four polypeptides: three initiate translation from non-AUG codons. Proc Natl Acad Sci USA 86:3978–3981

Florkiewicz RZ, Majack RA, Buechler RD, Florkiewicz E (1995) Quantitative export of FGF2 occurs through an alternative, energy-dependent, non-ER/Golgi pathway. J Cell Physiol 162:388–399

Floss T, Arnold HH, Braun T (1997) A role for FGF6 in skeletal muscle regeneration. Genes Dev 11:2040–2051

Galdemard C, Brison O, Lavialle C (1995) The proto-oncogene FGF3 is constitutively expressed in tumorigenic, but not in non-tumorigenic, clones of a human colon carcinoma cell line. Oncogene 10:2331–2342

Galzie Z, Kinsella AR, Smith JA (1997) Fibroblast growth factors and their receptors. Biochem Cell Biol 75:669–685

Gemel J, Gorry M, Ehrlich GD, MacArthur CA (1996) Structure and sequence of human FGF8. Genomics 35:253–257

Gospodarowicz D, Cheng J (1986) Heparin protects basic and acidic FGF from inactivation. J Cell Physiol 128:475–484

Grass S, Arnold HH, Braun T (1996) Alterations in somite patterning of Myf-5-deficient mice: a possible role for FGF4 and FGF6. Development 122:141–150

Halaban R, Kwon B, Ghosh S, Delli Bovi P, Baird A (1988) bFGF as an autocrine growth factor in human melanomas. Mol Cell Biol 8:2933–2941

Han J-K, Martin GR (1993) Embryonic expression of FGF6 is restricted to the skeletal muscle lineage. Dev Biol 158:549–554

Hartung H, Feldman B, Lovec H, Coulier F, Birnbaum D, Goldfarb M (1997) Murine FGF12 and FGF13: Expression in embryonic nervous system, connective tissue and heart. Mech Dev 64:31–39

Hattori Y, Yamasaki M, Konishi M, Itoh N (1997) Spatially restricted expression of fibroblast growth factor-10 mRNA in the rat brain. Mol Brain Res 47:139–146

Hecht D, Zimmerman N, Bedford M, Avivi A, Yayon A (1995) Identification of fibroblast growth factor 9 (FGF9) as a high affinity, heparin dependent ligand for FGF receptors 3 and 2 but not for FGF receptors 1 and 4. Growth Factors 12:223–233

Hoshikawa M, Ohbayashi N, Yonamine A, Konishi M, Ozaki K, Fukui S, Itoh N (1998) Structure and expression of a novel fibroblast growth factor, FGF17, preferentially expressed in the embryonic brain. Biochem Biophys Res Commun 244:187–191

Iida S, Yoshida T, Naito K et al (1992) Human hst-2 (FGF6) oncogene: cDNA cloning and characterization. Oncogene 7:303–309

Jaye M, Howk R, Burgess W et al (1986) Human endothelial cell growth factor: cloning, nucleotide sequence, and chromosome localization. Science 233:541–545

Keegan K, Rooke L, Hayman M, Spurr NK (1993) The fibroblast growth factor receptor 3 gene (FGFR3) is assigned to human chromosome 4. Cytogenet Cell Genet 62:172–175

Klagsbrun M, Baird A (1991) A dual receptor system is required for basic fibroblast growth factor activity. Cell 67:229–231

Lovec H, Hartung H, Verdier AS et al (1997) Assignment of FGF13 to human chromosome band Xq21 by in situ hybridization. Cytogenet Cell Genet 76:183–184

Marics I, Adelaide J, Raybaud F et al (1989) Characterization of the HST-related FGF.6 gene, a new member of the fibroblast growth factor gene family. Oncogene 4:335–340

Matsumoto-Yoshitomi S, Habashita J, Nomura C, Kuroshima K, Kurokawa T (1997) Autocrine transformation by fibroblast growth factor 9 (FGF9) and its possible participation in human oncogenesis. Int J Cancer 71:442–450

Mattei MG, DeLapeyriere O, Bresnick J, Dickson C, Birnbaum D, Mason I (1995) Mouse Fgf7 (fibroblast growth factor 7 and Fgf8 (fibroblast growth factor 8) genes map to chromosomes 2 and 19 respectively. Mammalian Genome 6:196–197

McWhirter JR, Goulding M, Weiner JA, Chun J, Murre C (1997) A novel fibroblast growth factor gene expressed in the developing nervous system is a downstream target of the chimeric homeodomain oncoprotein E2A-Pbx1. Development 124:3221–3232

Mergia A, Eddy R, Abraham JA, Fiddes JC, Shows TB (1986) The genes for basic and acidic fibroblast growth factors are on different human chromosomes. Biochem Biophys Res Commun 138:644–651

Mignatti P, Rifkin DB (1991) Release of basic fibroblast growth factor, an angiogenic factor devoid of secretory signal sequence: a trivial phenomenon or a novel secretion mechanism? J Cell Biochem 47:201–207

Miki T, Fleming TP, Bottaro DP, Rubin JS, Ron D, Aaronson SA (1991) Expression cDNA cloning of the KGF receptor by creation of a transforming autocrine loop. Science 251:72–75

Miyake A, Konishi M, Martin FH et al (1998) Structure and expression of a novel member, FGF16, of the fibroblast growth factor family. Biochem Biophys Res Commun 243:148–152

Miyamoto M, Naruo K-I, Seko C, Matsumoto S, Kondo T, Kurokawa T (1993) Molecular cloning of a novel cytokine cDNA encoding the ninth member of the fibroblast growth factor family, which has a unique secretion property. Mol Cell Biol 13:4251–4259

Nguyen C, Roux D, Mattei M-G et al (1988) The FGF-related oncogenes hst and int.2, and the bcl.1 locus are contained within one megabase in band q13 of chromosome 11, while the fgf.5 oncogene maps to 4q21. Oncogene 3:703–708

Niswander L, Tickle C, Vogel A, Martin G (1994) Function of FGF4 in limb development. Mol Reprod Dev 39:83–89

Ornitz DM, Leder P (1992) Ligand specificity and heparin dependence of fibroblast growth factor receptors 1 and 3. J Biol Chem 267:16305–16311

Ornitz DM, Xu JS, Colvin JS et al (1996) Receptor specificity of the fibroblast growth factor family. J Biol Chem 271:15292–15297

Peters G, Brookes S, Smith R, Placzek M, Dickson C (1989) The mouse homologue of the hst/k-FGF gene is adjacent to int-2 and is activated by proviral insertion in some virally induced mammary tumors. Proc Natl Acad Sci USA 86:5678–5682

Prestrelski SJ, Fox GM, Arakawa T (1992) Binding of heparin to basic fibroblast growth factor induces a conformational change. Arch Biochem Biophys 293:314–319

Renaud F, el Yazidi I, Boilly-Marer Y, Courtois Y, Laurent M (1996) Expression and regulation by serum of multiple FGF1 mRNA in normal transformed, and malignant human mammary epithelial cells. Biochem Biophys Res Commun 219:679–685

Rosen A, Sevelda P, Klein M et al (1993) First experience with FGF3 (INT-2) amplification in women with epithelial ovarian cancer. Br J Cancer 67:1122–1125

Schmitt JF, Susil BJ,Hearn MTW (1996) Aberrant FGF2, FGF3, FGF4 and C-ERB-B2 gene copy number in human ovarian, breast and endometrial tumours. Growth Factors 13:19–35

Shiang R, Thompson LM, Zhu Y-Z et al (1994) Mutations in the transmembrane domain of FGFR3 cause the most common genetic form of dwarfism, achondroplasia. Cell 78:335–342

Smallwood PM, Munoz-Sanjuan I, Tong P et al (1996) Fibroblast growth factor (FGF) homologous factors: new members of the FGF family implicated in nervous system development. Proc Natl Acad Sci USA 93:9850–9857

Tagashira S, Harada H, Katsumata T, Itoh N, Nakatsuka M (1997) Cloning of mouse FGF10 and up-regulation of its gene expression during wound healing. Gene 197:399–404

Talarico D, Ittmann M, Balsari A, Delli-Bovi P, Basch RS, Basilico C (1990) Protection of mice against tumor growth by immunization with an oncogene-encoded growth factor. Proc Natl Acad Sci USA 87:4222–4225

Tanaka A, Miyamoto K, Minamino N et al (1992) Cloning and characterization of an androgen-induced growth factor essential for the androgen-dependent growth of mouse mammary carcinoma cells. Proc Natl Acad Sci USA 89:8928–8932

Verdier AS, Mattei MG, Lovec H et al (1997) Chromosomal mapping of two novel human FGF genes, FGF11 and FGF12. Genomics 40:151–154

Vlodavsky I, Folkman J, Sullivan R et al (1987) Endothelial cell-derived basic fibroblast growth factor: synthesis and deposition into subendothelial extracellular matrix. Proc Natl Acad Sci USA 84:2292–2296

Vlodavsky I, Bar-Shavit R, Ishai-Michaeli R, Bashkin P, Fuks Z (1991) Extracellular sequestration and release of fibroblast growth factor: a regulatory mechanism? Trends Biochem Sci 16:268–271

Vogel A, Rodriguez C, Izpisúa-Belmonte JC (1996) Involvement of FGF8 in initiation, outgrowth and patterning of the vertebrate limb. Development 122:1737–1750

Warrington JA, Bailey SK, Armstrong E et al (1992) A radiation hybrid map of 18 growth factor, growth factor receptor, hormone receptor, or neurotransmitter receptor genes on the distal region of the long arm of chromosome 5. Genomics 13:803–808

White RA, Dowler LL, Angeloni SV, Pasztor LM, MacArthur CA (1995) Assignment of FGF8 to human chromosome 10q25-q26: mutations in FGF8 may be responsible for some types of acrocephalosyndactyly linked to this region. Genomics 30:109–111

Wilkinson DG, Bhatt S, McMahon AP (1989) Expression pattern of the FGF-related proto-oncogene int-2 suggests multiple roles in fetal development. Development 105:131–136

Wilkinson DG, Peters G, Dickson C, McMahon AP (1988) Expression of the FGF-related proto-oncogene int-2 during gastrulation and neurulation in the mouse. EMBO J 7:691–695

Wood S, Schertzer M, Yaremko ML (1995) Sequence identity locates CEBPD and FGFR1 to mapped human loci within proximal 8p. Cytogenet Cell Genet 70:188–191

Yoshida T, Miyagawa K, Odagiri H et al (1987) Genomic sequence of hst, a transforming gene encoding a protein homologous to fibroblast growth factors and the int-2-encoded protein. Proc Natl Acad Sci USA 84:7305–7309

Zhan X, Bates B, Hu X, Goldfarb M (1988) The human FGF5 oncogene encodes a novel protein related to fibroblast growth factors. Mol Cell Biol 8:3487–3497

2 Integrins and Angiogenesis

K.S. Riddelle-Spencer, D.A. Cheresh

2.1 Mechanisms of Blood Vessel Formation

New blood vessel formation in previously avascular tissue occurs by one of two similar but distinct mechanisms: vasculogenesis or angiogenesis. In vasculogenesis, blood vessels develop by organizing angioblast precursor cells into columns that then differentiate into vessels with lumens. Angiogenesis involves the outgrowth or sprouting of new vasculature from larger, pre-existing blood vessels (Risau 1995). The formation of new blood vessels is involved in the normal physiological processes of embryonic development, female reproduction, and wound healing (Folkman 1995). However, unregulated angiogenesis plays a critical role in various pathological mechanisms such as solid tumor formation, metastasis, childhood hemangiomas, and psoriasis, as well as inflammation-related diseases such as rheumatoid arthritis, osteoarthritis, and ulcerative colitis (Folkman 1995). Solid cancerous tumors will

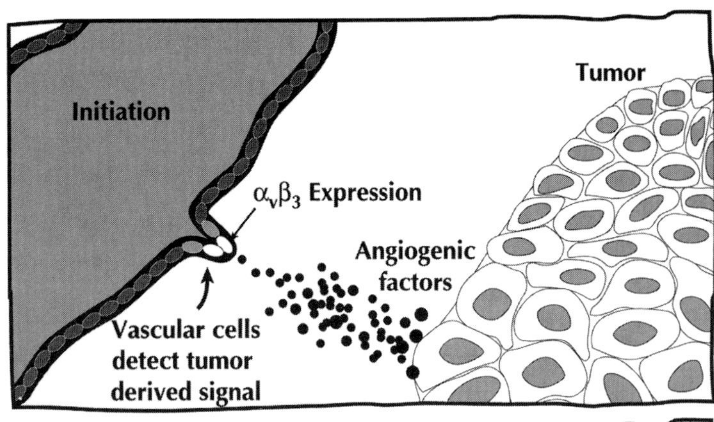
Tumor
Initiation
$\alpha_v\beta_3$ Expression
Angiogenic factors
Vascular cells detect tumor derived signal

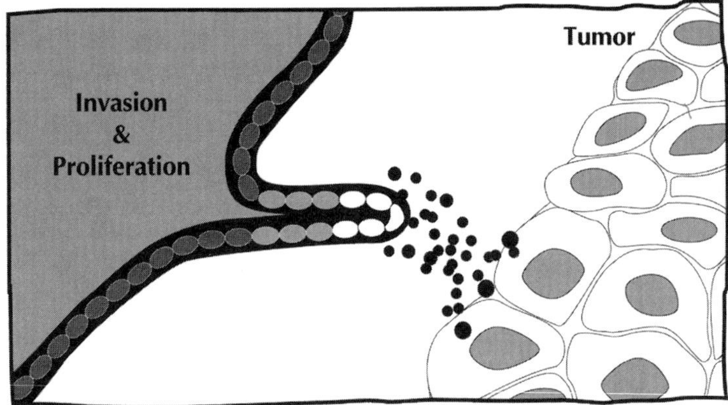
Tumor
Invasion & Proliferation

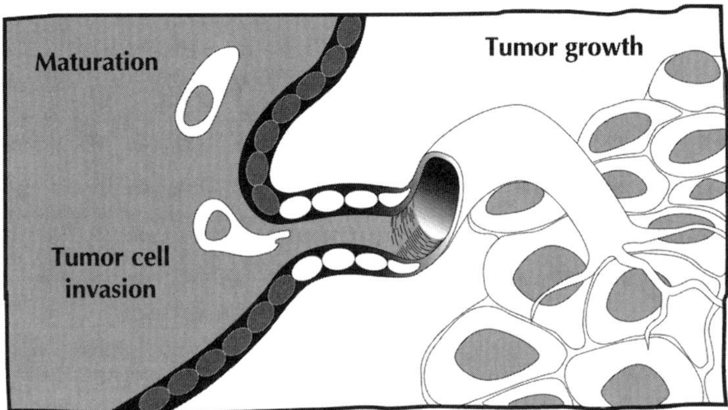
Maturation
Tumor growth
Tumor cell invasion

not expand beyond a minimal size unless new blood vessels supply oxygen, nutrients, and growth factors to the tumor cells (Folkman 1995). In addition, inappropriate vascularization of ocular tissues can lead to blindness; blood vessel growth into the normally avascular cornea can induce scarring, and proliferative vessels in the retina, as in diabetic retinopathy and macular degeneration, can induce retinal detachment and hemorrhage. Angiogenesis is also crucial for the formation of metastases at secondary sites by providing an avenue for metastatic cells to travel throughout the body. Therefore, a high degree of vascularization in certain tumors indicates an increased risk of metastasis and poor clinical prognosis (Weidner 1995). Hence, inhibitors or modulators of angiogenesis could be used for treatment of the diseases mentioned above.

The angiogenic process can be divided into three phases: initiation, proliferation/invasion, and maturation (Fig. 1). First, angiogenic stimulators, such as growth factors or cytokines, can be released from tumors and/or inflammatory cells. A number of angiogenic stimulators have been identified, such as basic fibroblast growth factor (bFGF), transforming growth factor alpha (TGF-α), and vascular endothelial growth factor (VEGF). These factors diffuse toward pre-existing blood vessels. Second, these angiogenic signals trigger the proliferation/invasion phase of angiogenesis, in which the endothelial cells secrete components of the extracellular matrix (ECM). The vascular cell receptors for bFGF,

◄

Fig. 1. Tumor-induced angiogenesis. Angiogenesis, the formation of new blood vessels from pre-existing vessels, can generally be divided into three phases, shown here in tumor-induced angiogenesis. First, angiogenic stimulators such as basic fibroblast growth factor (*bFGF*) and vascular endothelial growth factor (*VEGF*) are released from the tumor and/or inflammatory cells. These angiogenic signals trigger the invasion/proliferation phase, which is characterized by vascular cell proliferation, secretion of proteolytic enzymes and extracellular matrix (*ECM*) molecules, as well as altered expression of adhesion molecules. The proteolytic enzymes act to degrade ECM proteins, which, together with new synthesis of ECM molecules, results in remodeling of the extracellular microenvironment. The remodeling is crucial since it serves to facilitate vascular cell survival, proliferation and migration, resulting in a vascular invasion of the ECM. The maturation phase involves shape changes of the endothelial cells to achieve the final differentiated luminal structure in contact with a newly synthesized basement membrane (Stromblad and Cheresh 1996)

TGF-α, and VEGF are specific transmembrane receptors that become phosphorylated on tyrosine residues upon ligation. These events initiate signal transduction cascades, such as mitogen-activated protein (MAP)-kinase (ERK) pathways, which in turn promote changes in gene expression. In addition, the cells also produce proteolytic enzymes, which serve to remodel the extracellular microenvironment, making it more suitable for cell invasion. Growth factors and other angiogenic stimulators associated with the ECM can also be released upon matrix proteolysis, further enhancing the stimulatory effect. The endothelial cells invade the remodeled ECM and proliferate, thereby forming a sprout. This is accompanied by changes in the adhesive properties of the vascular cells, enabling them to respond to and interact with the remodeled ECM, ensuring continued cell survival, proliferation, and invasion. Finally, as cell differentiation and lumen formation occur, the vascular sprouts begin to mature. The new vessel secretes basement membrane components which serve to stabilize and maintain the endothelial cells in a differentiated and quiescent state. At this point, the new vessel can provide the tumor with nutrients while serving as a route for metastatic cells to leave the primary tumor and metastasize throughout the body.

2.2 Angiogenic Model Systems

Several model systems have been used to study the role of cell adhesion molecules in blood vessel formation. The most common in vivo models are the chick embryo chorioallantoic membrane (CAM), the rabbit corneal pocket, and the hamster cheek-pouch assay. In vivo models have also been developed in various other species, including mouse, rat, and quail; and there is also a human angiogenesis model using human skin transplanted onto the backs of severe combined immune deficient (SCID) mice (Bischoff 1995; Brooks et al. 1995; Drake et al. 1995). The strength of these models lies in the physiological coordination of complex processes for successful angiogenesis.

In addition, different in vitro models of capillary formation have been used to study growth of endothelial cells into matrix-containing gels or tubular formation in two dimensions (Bischoff 1995). Under such conditions, endothelial cells become quiescent and form tubular structures, which has been suggested as representing the terminal stage of angiogenesis, involving endothelial cell differentiation (Kubota et al. 1988). In addition, a model involving proliferative tubes derived from fragments of rat aorta invading a fibrin- or collagen-containing gel has also been developed (Nicosia and Madri 1987; Bischoff 1995). The strength of most of these in vitro models is that they are relatively easy to perform and represent well-defined experimental conditions. However, results obtained from these models must be considered to represent only a portion of the complex process of angiogenesis observed in vivo.

2.3 Extracellular Matrix and Angiogenesis

Adhesion between endothelial cells and the underlying ECM are involved in multiple steps of angiogenesis. During angiogenesis, dynamic remodeling of the ECM, involving both matrix degradation and deposition of new ECM components into the extracellular environment, takes place to facilitate the different phases of angiogenesis. For example, during wound healing in skin, as well as in retinal and intraembryonal vasculogenesis, fibronectin is deposited relatively early, followed by laminin, preceding the differentiation phase (Clark et al. 1982; Risau and Lemmon 1988; Jiang et al. 1994). However, among the ECM adhesive substrates, collagens are the matrix proteins best associated with angiogenesis in vivo. Ingber and Folkman demonstrated that inhibiting collagen deposition, triple helix formation, and cross-linking, prevented angiogenesis (Ingber 1991). This is supported by other studies demonstrating the requirement for collagen synthesis in angiogenesis (Hanemaaijer et al. 1993; Haralabopoulos et al. 1994). Also, targeted gene knockout of the collagen type I α1-chain caused rupture of blood vessels, indicating defects in early blood vessel development (Lohler et al. 1984).

Both collagen deposition and its degradation are required for angiogenesis. Degradation of collagen is mediated, at least in part, by matrix metalloproteinases (MMPs), which are regulated at the level of gene expression and enzymatic activity. MMPs can be converted from inert to the active form by proteolysis, a process that is inhibited by the presence of tissue inhibitors of metalloproteinases (TIMPs). Different angiogenic stimulators, such as bFGF, phorbol-12-myristate-13-acetate (PMA), and tumor necrosis factor α (TNF-α), stimulate endothelial cell expression of MMPs (Takigawa et al. 1990; Moses et al. 1990). This induction may be important during angiogenesis, since inhibition of MMPs by TIMP-1, TIMP-2, and an MMP inhibitor from cartilage has been found to block angiogenesis in the chick embryo yolk sac, chick CAM, and rat cornea models (Moses et al. 1990; Takigawa et al. 1990; Johnson et al. 1994).

The fact that both de novo collagen synthesis and collagen proteolysis are involved in angiogenesis may at first appear contradictory, but temporal regulation of these events may be crucial when considering the distinct matrix microenvironments necessary during various phases of angiogenesis. The invasive phase includes degradation of both the basement membrane and the surrounding stroma, which facilitates cell proliferation and migration. Eliminating a quiescence signal from the basement membrane may bring this about, since an intact basement membrane tends to maintain differentiated endothelium. Stromal collagen breakdown may also expose cryptic adhesive sites. These sites in collagen could provide a provisional matrix for the endothelial cells during this phase of angiogenesis. This demonstrates how adhesive and proteolytic mechanisms might be coordinated during the process of angiogenesis. The synthesis and deposition of a new basement membrane including collagen type IV and laminin may then facilitate differentiation during the latter stages of angiogenesis (Ingber 1991). These studies demonstrate a role for ECM-cellular interactions, suggesting a direct association of signaling and cell survival events with cell adhesion receptors such as integrins.

2.4 Integrins

The various angiogenic phases of vascular endothelial cells are regulated by one or more members of the integrin family of cell adhesion receptors (Brooks et al. 1994a,b). The integrin family is composed of over 15 alpha and 8 beta subunits that are expressed in over 20 different $\alpha\beta$ heterodimeric combinations on cell surfaces. Integrins are a family of heterodimeric transmembrane adhesion receptors mediating cell-ECM interactions and, in some cases, cell-cell adhesion (Hynes 1992). In addition, integrins also mediate transmembrane signaling from the ECM into the cell, as well as reorganize the cytoskeleton to facilitate cell migration (Clark and Brugge 1995; Yamada and Miyamoto 1995). Multiple integrins are expressed on endothelial cells, allowing attachment to a wide spectrum of ECM components (Cheng and Kramer 1989). For example, collagen types I and IV both contain cryptic RGD (Arg-Gly-Asp) sequences that can be recognized by integrin αvβ3 only after proteolysis of the intact collagen triple helix (Davis 1992; Pfaff et al. 1993; Montgomery et al. 1994). In fact, αvβ3 integrin is expressed on vascular cells preferentially during the proliferative and invasive phases of angiogenesis (Brooks et al. 1994a, b).

Targeted gene knockout studies in mice point to the importance of a fibronectin receptor, integrin α5, in blood vessel development in vivo. Knockout of α5 resulted in multiple lethal defects in early embryonic development, including defective blood vessel formation similar to what is observed in fibronectin knockouts (Watt and Hodivala 1994). However, integrin function during blood vessel formation in vivo has been studied most extensively for αvβ3 (Brooks et al. 1994a). The integrin αvβ3 is a receptor for a wide variety of extracellular matrix proteins with an exposed tripeptide Arg-Gly-Asp (RGD) (Cheresh 1993). αvβ3 mediates cellular adhesion to vitronectin, fibronectin, fibrinogen, laminin, collagen, von Willebrand factor, osteopontin, and adenovirus penton base, among others (Cheresh 1987, 1993; Leavesley et al. 1992). Thus, expression of this integrin enables a cell to adhere to, migrate on, or respond to almost any matrix protein. Despite its behavior, αvβ3 is not widely expressed and not readily detectable in quiescent blood vessels. However, this receptor appears most prominently on cytokine-activated endothelial cells. For example, basic fibroblast growth factor (bFGF), but not TGF-beta or interferon gamma, markedly increase β3 mRNA and surface expression in cultured human dermal microvascular endothelial cells (Enenstein et al. 1992; Sepp et al. 1994). Basic FGF and TNF-α stimulate αvβ3 expression on developing blood vessels in the CAM (Brooks et al. 1994b) and on the rabbit cornea (Friedlander et al. 1995). Upregulation of αvβ3 expression is also induced by human tumors cultured on the CAM (Brooks et al. 1994a,b), by human tumors grown in human skin explants grafted onto SCID mice, and in the rabbit cornea. Integrin αvβ3 also is significantly upregulated on vascular cells in vivo during wound healing (Brooks et al. 1994b), macular degeneration, diabetic retinopathy, and other neovascular diseases of the eye (unpublished observations).

Integrin αvβ3 is not a prerequisite for blood vessel development, since patients suffering from a form of Glanzmann's thrombasthenia have apparently normal blood vessels despite either lacking the β3 subunit or expressing a mutant nonfunctional version (Coller et al. 1991; Djaffar and Rosa 1993). However, these individuals are severely deficient in their wound repair function. Patients with this disorder may develop blood vessels in the absence of αvβ3, owing to an alternative mechanism involving integrin αvβ3, which potentiates a distinct pathway of angiogenesis (Friedlander et al. 1995), as described below.

Vascular cells also express a wide variety of integrin adhesion receptors (Cheresh 1987; Cheresh et al. 1989; Leavesley et al. 1993; Enenstein and Kramer 1994). In fact, a number of vascular cell integrins are functionally and structurally homologous, suggesting some level of redundancy. Hence, in addition to the influence of αvβ3, the functionally homologous integrin αvβ5 also has a role in angiogenesis. In bFGF-stimulated angiogenesis, antagonists to αvβ3, but not αvβ5, were able to reduce new blood vessel growth significantly in both the rabbit cornea and chick CAM models. However, in VEGF-induced angiogenesis, only the αvβ5 antagonists, not those directed toward αvβ3, affected angiogenesis (Friedlander et al. 1995). That αvβ5 functions in VEGF-induced angiogenesis may be clinically relevant, as VEGF is reported to be associated with ischemia-induced ocular angiogenesis (Miller et al. 1994), and is increased in intraocular fluids obtained from patients with active neovascular disease (Aiello et al. 1994).

2.5 Integrins, Cell Survival, and Apoptosis

The highly restricted expression of αvβ3 and its upregulation during angiogenesis suggest that it may play a critical role in the angiogenic process. In fact, recent experimental evidence supports this notion. Specifically, disruption of αvβ3 ligation to its ECM by antibody or peptide antagonists of αvβ3 prevents blood vessel formation in the chick CAM, quail embryo, rabbit cornea, mouse retina, and in human skin transplanted onto SCID mice (Brooks et al. 1995; Drake et al. 1995; Friedlander et al. 1995; Hammes et al. 1996). Angiogenic vascular cells exposed to antibody against αvβ3 selectively become apoptotic, indicating that this antibody blocks vascular proliferation by inducing these proliferating endothelial cells to undergo unscheduled apoptosis (Brooks et al. 1994b). This suggests that integrin αvβ3 has a unique function during angiogenesis, namely to provide specific survival signals that eventually facilitate vascular cell proliferation.

Several investigators have focused on the relationship between cell adhesion and vascular cell survival. Using the chick CAM model, Eliceiri et al. demonstrated the dependence of both αvβ3 and growth factor receptor ligation in promoting angiogenesis through signaling events. When stimulated with bFGF, two endothelial cell mitogen-activated protein (MAP)-kinase (ERK) signals are activated: one immediate and integrin-independent; and another αvβ3-dependent signal maintained for several hours (Eliceiri et al. 1998). This suggests that angiogenesis depends on sustained ERK activity regulated by both a growth factor receptor and integrin αvβ3. ERK activation has been implicated in cell survival (Xia 1995). Furthermore, primary endothelial cells are anchorage-dependent and undergo apoptosis when denied integrin-mediated attachment (Meredith et al. 1993; Re et al. 1994). Re and colleagues related endothelial cell survival to the degree of cell spreading on fibronectin and vitronectin, implicating reorganization of the cytoskeleton as an important factor for endothelial cell survival (Re et al. 1994). Taken together, these studies indicated that integrins regulate endothelial cell survival in vitro. However, the particular integrin mediating cell survival might be cell-type- and -condition-specific. This may in part be explained by the distinct roles of different extracellular matrix components. For example, provisional matrices, such as fibronectin, vitronectin, and fibrinogen, typically potentiate cell proliferation, whereas the basement membrane, i.e., laminin and collagen IV, promotes cell cycle withdrawal and differentiation (Adams and Watt 1993; Lin and Bissell 1993). Therefore, attachment to different ECM components is mediated through specific integrins that can generate distinct signals to promote cell survival in multiple ways.

As described above, blocking αvβ3 resulted in unscheduled apoptosis among proliferating vascular cells (Brooks et al. 1994b). Specific antibody or cyclic peptide antagonists of αvβ3 administered during angiogenesis in the chick CAM also induced endothelial cell p53-dependent DNA-binding activity, whereas antibodies to β1 had no effect on p53 activity or apoptosis (Brooks et al. 1994b; Stromblad et al. 1996). Ligation of αvβ3 also enhanced Bcl-2 expression while decreasing that of Bax. The resulting increase in the Bcl-2:Bax ratio has previously been shown to promote cell survival (White 1996). αvβ3 binding to ECM appears, therefore, to suppress apoptosis and conflicting growth arrest signals, thereby facilitating proliferation and maturation of new blood vessels during angiogenesis.

2.6 Matrix Metalloproteinase-2

As mentioned above, integrin αvβ3 is known to bind a number of ECM proteins. More recent studies show that integrin αvβ3 can also bind directly to the C-terminus of the proteolytically active matrix metalloproteinase-2 (MMP-2) (Fig. 2), thus localizing the MMP-2-mediated matrix degradation capacity at the invasive/migratory vascular cell site during angiogenesis (Brooks et al. 1996). Several lines of evidence support this. Firstly, αvβ3 and MMP-2 were localized on the surface of invasive angiogenic vascular cells and melanoma cells in vivo. Secondly, direct interaction between αvβ3 and MMP-2 was demonstrated between these proteins in vitro. It is of interest that MMP-2 does not contain an RGD sequence and, therefore, it is not clear how αvβ3

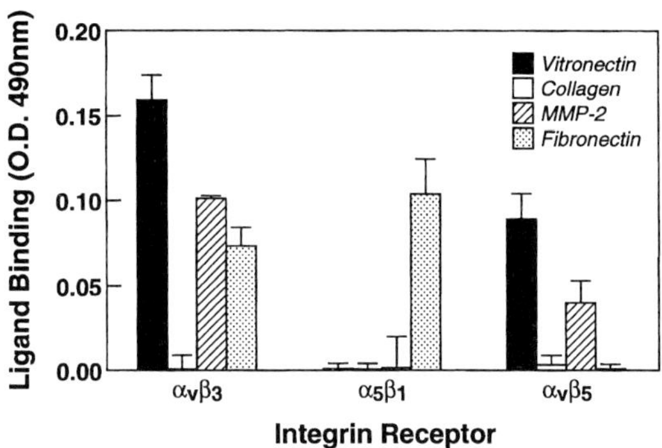

Fig. 2. Purified integrin receptors (1 μg/ml), αvβ3, αvβ5, and α5β1 were coated on wells of a 96-well microtiter plate. Integrin ligands, including vitronectin, collagen, and fibronectin or purified recombinant MMP-2 (5 ng) were incubated in wells coated with integrin receptors. Specific protein binding was quantified by measuring reactivity of ligand-specific antibodies. Data bars represent the mean plus or minus standard error of ligand binding from three to five experiments with triplicate wells (Brooks et al. 1996)

interacts with MMP-2. Finally, expression of αvβ3 on cultured CS-1 melanoma cells enabled them to bind soluble recombinant MMP-2, facilitating collagen degradation. In addition, MMP-2 inhibited β3 expressing CS-1 cell attachment to vitronectin. However, these cells could attach and spread on immobilized type IV collagen in the presence of active cell-surface-associated MMP-2. These findings suggest that αvβ3 can simultaneously bind both MMP-2 and proteolyzed collagen fragments. Interestingly, while αvβ3 fails to bind native collagen, it does interact with proteolyzed collagen due to exposure of cryptic RGD sites (Davis 1992; Montgomery et al. 1994), suggesting that αvβ3 on the surface of invasive cells can both regulate collagen degradation and interact with the resulting fragments. In fact, this is supported by the observation that αvβ3 antagonists (Brooks et al. 1994b; Brooks et al. 1995), as well as TIMPs, block angiogenesis in vivo (Moses et al. 1990). Therefore, it is possible that αvβ3 and MMP-2 functionally cooperate to promote the invasive behavior of angiogenic vascular cells.

2.7 PEX – A Natural Inhibitor of Angiogenesis

Recently, it has been shown that a naturally occurring fragment of MMP-2 prevents intact MMP-2 from binding to αvβ3 (Brooks et al. 1998). This fragment, termed PEX, comprises the noncatalytic C-terminal hemopexin-like domain of MMP-2. PEX is a naturally occurring MMP-2 breakdown product that can inhibit cell-associated collagenolytic activity both in vitro and in vivo (Fig. 3). Importantly, PEX can be detected in vivo in tumors and during developmental retinal neovascularization. Levels of PEX in these vascularized tissues suggest that it interacts with endothelial cell αvβ3 to serve as a natural inhibitor of MMP-2 activity, regulating the invasive behavior of new blood vessels. These findings are consistent with previously reported results indicating that the hemopexin domain of MMP-2 prevents cell-mediated MMP-2 activation (Strongin et al. 1993; Zucker et al. 1995; Foda et al. 1996). Furthermore, systemic administration of recombinant PEX blocked collagenolytic activity in vivo, leading to a significant reduction in the growth of CS-1 melanoma tumors grown on the CAM model (Brooks et al. 1998). The effect was related to its capacity to reduce angiogenesis significantly in these tumors. Importantly, these CS-1

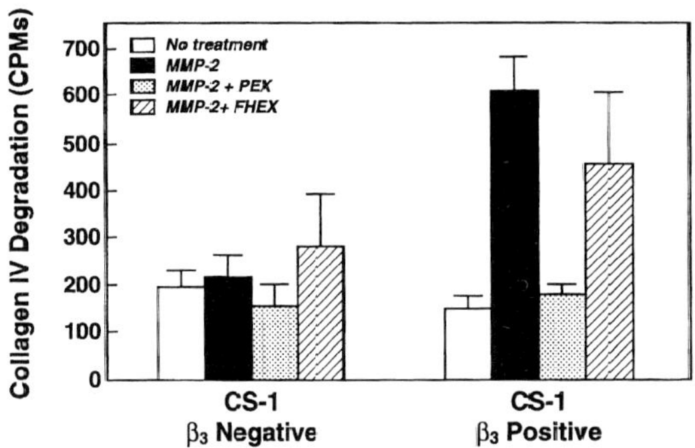

Fig. 3. Cell-mediated collagen degradation by CS-1 melanoma cells. In a typical experiment, the collagenase activity was two- to threefold over background levels (Brooks et al. 1998)

melanoma tumors display no functional expression of integrin αvβ3 and produce little if any endogenous MMP-2, providing further evidence that the observed inhibition of tumor growth is due to suppression of tumor-associated angiogenesis. In fact, PEX did not influence the growth rate of CS-1 cells in vitro, supporting the notion that the anti-tumor activity of PEX is due to its anti-angiogenic effects. The fact that PEX blocks αvβ3-directed MMP-2 activity and disrupts angiogenesis suggests that PEX accumulation during blood vessel maturation provides a feedback mechanism to prevent inappropriate blood vessel sprouting.

These findings illustrate a novel cell biological mechanism accounting for the regulation of extracellular matrix remodeling which influences cellular invasion events critical for angiogenesis. In this case, integrin αvβ3 likely serves two functions. Firstly, it binds to MMP-2, facilitating collagenase activity important for cell invasion (Brooks et al. 1996). This likely depends on the ability of αvβ3 to bind selectively proteolyzed fragments of collagen, leading to signals required for cell survival (Montgomery et al. 1994). Secondly, αvβ3 facilitates cleavage of MMP-2 and accumulation of a noncatalytic fragment (PEX) that inhibits cell invasion. Accordingly, the appearance of PEX at sites of neovascularization may serve not only to control normal angiogenesis or neovascularization but, when administered exogenously, also to provide a therapeutic inhibitor of diseases associated with angiogenesis.

2.8 Future Perspectives

Angiogenesis is a very complex process involving regulation of vascular cell survival, proliferation, migration, differentiation, and maturation. Many of these events depend on vascular cell adhesion potentiated by both cell-cell and cell-matrix interactions. It is becoming clear that specific antagonists of certain cell adhesion events may influence various steps in the angiogenic cascade. Future studies will determine whether such antagonists prove useful in humans, where they may influence diseases associated with angiogenesis such as cancer, diabetic retinopathy, and various inflammatory disorders.

References

Adams JC, Watt FM (1993) Regulation of development and differentiation by the extracellular matrix. Development 117(4):1183–1198

Aiello LP, Avery RL, Arrigg PG, et al (1994) Vascular endothelial growth factor in ocular fluid of patients with diabetic retinopathy and other retinal disorders (see comments). N Engl J Med 331:1480–1487

Bischoff J (1995) Approaches to studying cell adhesion molecules in angiogenesis. Trends Cell Biol 5:69–74

Brooks PC, Clark RA, Cheresh DA (1994a) Requirement of vascular integrin alpha v beta 3 for angiogenesis. Science 264(5158):569–571

Brooks PC, Montgomery AM, Rosenfeld M, et al (1994b) Integrin alpha v beta 3 antagonists promote tumor regression by inducing apoptosis of angiogenic blood vessels. Cell 79(7):1157–1164

Brooks PC, Stromblad S, et al (1995) Antiintegrin alpha v beta 3 blocks human breast cancer growth and angiogenesis in human skin (see comments). J Clin Invest 96(4):1815–1822

Brooks PC, Stromblad S, Sanders LC, et al (1996) Localization of matrix metalloproteinase MMP-2 to the surface of invasive cells by interaction with integrin alpha v beta 3. Cell 85(5):683–693

Brooks PC, Silletti S, Schalscha TL von, et al (1998) Disruption of angiogenesis by PEX, a noncatalytic metalloproteinase fragment with integrin binding activity. Cell 92(3):391–400

Cheng YF, Kramer RH (1989) Human microvascular endothelial cells express integrin-related complexes that mediate adhesion to the extracellular matrix. J Cell Physiol 139(2):275–286

Cheresh DA (1987) Human endothelial cells synthesize and express an Arg-Gly-Asp-directed adhesion receptor involved in attachment to fibrinogen and von Willebrand factor. Proc Natl Acad Sci USA 84(18):6471–6475

Cheresh DA (1993) Integrins: structure, function, and biological properties. Adv Mol Cell Biol 6:225–252

Cheresh DA, Berliner SA, Vicente V, Ruggeri ZM (1989) Recognition of distinct adhesive sites on fibrinogen by related integrins on platelets and endothelial cells. Cell 58(5):945–953

Clark EA, Brugge JS (1995) Integrins and signal transduction pathways: the road taken. Science 268(5208):233–239

Clark RA, DellaPelle P, Manseau E, et al (1982) Blood vessel fibronectin increases in conjunction with endothelial cell proliferation and capillary ingrowth during wound healing. J Invest Dermatol 79(5):269–276

Coller BS, Cheresh DA, Asch E, Seligsohn U (1991) Platelet vitronectin receptor expression differentiates Iraqi-Jewish from Arab patients with Glanzmann thrombasthenia in Israel. Blood 77(1):75–83

Davis GE (1992) Affinity of integrins for damaged extracellular matrix: alpha v beta 3 binds to denatured collagen type I through RGD sites. Biochem Biophys Res Commun 182(3):1025–1031

Djaffar I, Rosa JP (1993) A second case of variant of Glanzmann's thrombasthenia due to substitution of platelet GPIIIa (integrin beta 3) Arg214 by Trp. Hum Mol Genet 2(12):2179–2180

Drake CJ, Cheresh DA, Little CD (1995) An antagonist of integrin alpha v beta 3 prevents maturation of blood vessels during embryonic neovascularization. J Cell Sci 108(7):2655–2661

Eliceiri BP, Klemke R, Stromblad S, Cheresh DA (1998) Integrin alpha v beta3 requirement for sustained mitogen-activated protein kinase activity during angiogenesis. J Cell Biol 140(5):1255–1263

Enenstein J, Kramer RH (1994) Confocal microscopic analysis of integrin expression on the microvasculature and its sprouts in the neonatal foreskin. J Invest Dermatol 103(3):381–386

Enenstein J, Waleh NS, Kramer RH (1992) Basic FGF and TGF-beta differentially modulate integrin expression of human microvascular endothelial cells. Exp Cell Res 203(2):499–503

Foda HD, George S, et al (1996) Activation of human umbilical vein endothelial cell progelatinase A by phorbol myristate acetate: a protein kinase C-dependent mechanism involving a membrane-type matrix metalloproteinase. Lab Invest 74(2):538–545

Folkman J(1995) Angiogenesis in cancer, vascular, rheumatoid and other disease. Nat Med 1(1):27–31

Friedlander, M, Brooks PC, et al (1995) Definition of two angiogenic pathways by distinct alpha v integrins. Science 270(5241):1500–1502

Hammes HP, Brownlee M, Jonczyk A, et al (1996) Subcutaneous injection of a cyclic peptide antagonist of vitronectin receptor-type integrins inhibits retinal neovascularization. Nat Med 2(5):529–533

Hanemaaijer R, Koolwijk P, le Clercq L, et al (1993) Regulation of matrix metalloproteinase expression in human vein and microvascular endothelial cells. Effects of tumour necrosis factor alpha, interleukin 1 and phorbol ester. Biochem J 296(3):803–809

Haralabopoulos GC, Grant DS, Kleinman HK, et al (1994) Inhibitors of basement membrane collagen synthesis prevent endothelial cell alignment in matrigel in vitro and angiogenesis in vivo. Lab Invest 71(4):575–582

Hynes RO (1992) Integrins: versatility, modulation, and signaling in cell adhesion. Cell 69(1):11–25

Ingber D (1991) Extracellular matrix and cell shape: potential control points for inhibition of angiogenesis. J Cell Biochem 47(3):236–241

Jiang B, Liou GI, Behzadian MA, et al (1994) Astrocytes modulate retinal vasculogenesis: effects on fibronectin expression. J Cell Sci 107(9):2499–2508

Johnson MD, Kim HR, Chesler L, et al (1994) Inhibition of angiogenesis by tissue inhibitor of metalloproteinase. J Cell Physiol 160(1):194–202

Kubota Y, Kleinman HK, Martin GR, et al (1988) Role of laminin and basement membrane in the morphological differentiation of human endothelial cells into capillary-like structures. J Cell Biol 107(4):1589–1598

Leavesley DI, Ferguson GD, Wayner EA, Cheresh DA (1992) Requirement of the integrin beta 3 subunit for carcinoma cell spreading or migration on vitronectin and fibrinogen. J Cell Biol 117(5):1101–1107

Leavesley DI, Schwartz MA, Rosenfeld M, Cheresh DA (1993) Integrin beta 1- and beta 3-mediated endothelial cell migration is triggered through distinct signaling mechanisms. J Cell Biol 121(1):163–170

Lin CQ, Bissell MJ (1993) Multi-faceted regulation of cell differentiation by extracellular matrix (see comments). Faseb J 7(9):737–743

Lohler J, Timpl R, Jaenisch R (1984) Embryonic lethal mutation in mouse collagen I gene causes rupture of blood vessels and is associated with erythropoietic and mesenchymal cell death. Cell 38(2):597–607

Meredith JE Jr, Fazeli B, Schwartz MA (1993) The extracellular matrix as a cell survival factor. Mol Biol Cell 4(9):953–961

Miller JW, Adamis AP, Shima DT, et al (1994) Vascular endothelial growth factor/vascular permeability factor is temporally and spatially correlated with ocular angiogenesis in a primate model. Am J Pathol 145(3):574–584

Montgomery AM, Reisfeld RA, Cheresh DA (1994) Integrin alpha v beta 3 rescues melanoma cells from apoptosis in three-dimensional dermal collagen. Proc Natl Acad Sci USA 91(19):8856–8860

Moses MA, Sudhalter J, Langer R (1990) Identification of an inhibitor of neovascularization from cartilage. Science 248(4961):1408–1410

Nicosia RF, Madri JA (1987) The microvascular extracellular matrix. Developmental changes during angiogenesis in the aortic ring-plasma clot model. Am J Pathol 128(1):78–90

Pfaff M, Aumailley M, Specks U, et al (1993) Integrin and Arg-Gly-Asp dependence of cell adhesion to the native and unfolded triple helix of collagen type VI. Exp Cell Res 206(1):167–176

Re F, Zanetti A, Sironi N, et al (1994) Inhibition of anchorage-dependent cell spreading triggers apoptosis in cultured human endothelial cells. J Cell Biol 127(2):537–546

Risau W(1995) Differentiation of endothelium. FASEB J 9(10):926–933

Risau W, Lemmon V (1988) Changes in the vascular extracellular matrix during embryonic vasculogenesis and angiogenesis. Dev Biol 125(2):441–450

Sepp NT, Li L-J, Lee KH, Brown EJ, Caughman SWW, Lawley TJ, Swerlick RA (1994) Basic fibroblast growth factor increases expression of the $\alpha v\beta 3$ complex on human microvessel endothelial cells. J Invest Dermatol 103:295–299

Stromblad S, Cheresh DA (1996) Cell adhesion and angiogenesis. Trends Cell Biol 6:462–468

Stromblad S, Becker JC, Yebra M, et al (1996) Suppression of p53 activity and p21WAF1/CIP1 expression by vascular cell integrin alphaVbeta3 during angiogenesis. J Clin Invest 98(2):426–433

Strongin AY, Marmer BL, Grant GA, Goldberg GI (1993) Plasma membrane-dependent activation of the 72-kDa type IV collagenase is prevented by complex formation with TIMP-2. J Biol Chem 268(19):14033–14039

Takigawa M, Nishida Y, Suzuki F, et al (1990) Induction of angiogenesis in chick yolk-sac membrane by polyamines and its inhibition by tissue inhibitors of metalloproteinases (TIMP and TIMP-2). Biochem Biophys Res Commun 171(3):1264–1271

Watt FM, Hodivala KJ (1994) Cell adhesion. Fibronectin and integrin knockouts come unstuck. Curr Biol 4(3):270–272

Weidner N (1995) Intratumor microvessel density as a prognostic factor in cancer (comment). Am J Pathol 147(1):9–19

White E (1996) Life, death, and the pursuit of apoptosis. Genes Dev 10(1):1–15

Xia Z, Dickens M, Raingeaud J, Davis RJ, Greenberg ME (1995) Opposing effects of ERK and JNK-p38 MAP kinases on apoptosis. Science 270(5240):1326–1331

Yamada KM, Miyamoto S (1995) Integrin transmembrane signaling and cytoskeletal control. Curr Opin Cell Biol 7(5):681–689

Zucker S, Conner C, et al (1995) Thrombin induces the activation of progelatinase A in vascular endothelial cells. Physiologic regulation of angiogenesis. J Biol Chem 270(40):23730–23738

3 Mechanisms of Brain Angiogenesis in Health and Disease

K.H. Plate

3.1 Introduction

The vascular system is responsible for supplying all organs in a body with blood, oxygen and nutrients and for removing waste products. As a reflection of this highly important function, the vascular system is the first organ system to be formed in a mammalian embryo. Thereafter, the growth of all organs is accompanied by a similar expansion of the vascular system.

3.2 Angiogenesis in Normal Brain

During development, the brain is vascularized by capillary sprouts which originate from the primitive perineural vascular plexus. The onset of angiogenesis occurs during a certain stage of embryonic development (e.g., on E4.5 during chick embryonic development and E11 in the mouse), is maximal in the early postnatal period, and downregulated in the adult brain (Risau 1995). From these observations, the hypothesis has been proposed that the developing brain produces an angiogenesis factor to stimulate proliferation of endothelial cells and attract them chemotactically. There is considerable evidence that VEGF is a major regulator of embryonic angiogenesis (for review see Risau 1997). This hypothesis is supported by the following observations:

1. The spatial and temporal expression patterns of VEGF mRNA and its high affinity receptors VEGF receptor 1 (VEGF-R1) (flt-1) and VEGF receptor 2 (VEGF-R2) (KDR/flk-1) correspond to angiogenesis during mouse embryonic development.
2. VEGF mRNA is expressed in the ventricular layer of the developing neuroectoderm, which corresponds to the area of directed ingrowth of blood vessels from the perineural vascular plexus (Breier et al. 1992).
3. VEGF-R1 and -R2, on the other hand, are expressed by blood vessels of the vascular plexus and capillaries that have invaded the neuroectoderm (Millauer et al. 1993; Breier et al. 1995; Dumont et al. 1995).

The family of VEGF genes has recently been considerably expanded (Table 1). Null mice have been developed for placenta growth factor (PlGF), which binds to VEGF-R1 and for VEGF-B, which also binds to VEGF-R1 (G. Persico and U. Eriksson, unpublished observations). Both mice are viable without obvious vascular phenotypes, arguing against a critical role for PlGF and VEGF-B in vascular development.

Recently, two additional endothelial cell-specific receptor tyrosine kinases, tie1 (tie) and tie2 (tek), have been described. These belong to a novel class of transmembrane receptors whose extracellular domains are characterized by an unusual array of immunoglobulin (Ig)-like domains, epidermal growth factor (EGF) -like repeats, and fibronectin type III repeats. Tie1 and tie2 are expressed early in the development of the vascular system and appear to be coexpressed by most blood vessels and capillaries (Dumont et al. 1992, 1995; Schnürch and Risau 1993; Maisonpierre et al. 1993). High mRNA levels are observed in the vasculature of the developing brain (Schnürch and Risau 1993; Dumont

Table 1. Currently identified endothelial cell specific receptor/ligand systems

Receptor	VEGF-R1	VEGF-R2	VEGF-R3	Tie1	Tie2
Ligand(s)	VEGF VEGF-B PIGF	VEGF VEGF-C VEGF-D VEGF-E	VEGF-C VEGF-D	?	Ang-1 Ang-2 Ang-3 Ang-4

VEGF, VEGF-R1, VEGF-R2, tie1, tie2, and angiopoietin-1 and -2 are essential for normal vascular development in mice (see Carmeliet et al. 1996; Ferrara et al. 1996; Fong et al. 1995; Shalaby et al. 1995; Sato et al. 1995; Suri et al. 1996; Maisonpierre et al. 1997). VEGF-B- and PIGF-knockout mice develop normally, arguing against a critical role of these growth factors in embryonic blood vessel development.

et al. 1995). Consistent with a possible role in brain angiogenesis, tie1 and tie2 are downregulated in the adult organism. Knockouts of the *tie1* and *tie2* genes in transgenic mice have shown that both receptors are essential for normal vascular development, but displayed a distinct phenotype in VEGF-R-null mice. Tie-deficient mice die later during embryonic development or after birth and show phenotypical alterations consistent with a role in vascular remodeling (Dumont et al. 1994; Sato et al. 1995; Puri et al. 1995). These findings recently have been considerably expanded by the cloning of two tie2 ligands, angiopoietin-1 and -2. Ang-1-null mice showed defects reminiscent of the tie2 knockout, suggesting that Ang-1 is a physiological ligand for tie2 in vivo. Overexpression of Angiopoietin-2, which blocks Ang-1-mediated tie2 signaling, lead to a similar phenotype (Davis et al. 1996; Suri et al. 1996; Maisonpierre et al. 1997).

3.3 Angiogenesis in Brain Tumor Development and Progression

It has been proposed for several decades that angiogenesis is an intrinsic part of tumor development and progression (see Folkman 1990). On the other hand, inhibition of tumor angiogenesis might be a viable approach to treating malignant tumors (Gimbrone et al. 1972; Folkman and

Hanahan 1991). These hypotheses are based on the following observations:

1. Tumor cells are able to secrete endothelial cell growth factors and induce angiogenesis in in vivo test systems such as the chorioallantoic membrane assay (Folkman 1990).
2. Malignant tumors are consistently better vascularized than their benign counterparts or precursor lesions, a phenomenon described as a "switch to the angiogenic state" (Hanahan and Folkman 1996).
3. Several compounds have been shown to inhibit endothelial cell proliferation in vitro and tumor growth in vivo (Moses and Langer 1991).

The molecular mechanisms underlying tumor angiogenesis have only been discovered in part. Evidence is accumulating, however, that molecules regulating blood vessel growth and differentiation under physiological conditions (e.g., in the developing embryo) are similarly involved in regulation of tumor angiogenesis.

We have investigated the role of VEGF and its receptors, and, more recently, the role of angiopoietins and TIE receptors in tumor angiogenesis (for review see Plate et al. 1994a; Plate and Risau 1995; Breier et al. 1997) using malignant gliomas as a model system. Malignant gliomas are neuroectodermal tumors which most commonly arise in the white matter of the cerebral hemispheres. The most common glioma is called glioblastoma, a tumor characterized by highly polymorphic tumor cells, high proliferation of tumor cells, invasion of normal brain structures by migrating glioma cells, and induction of angiogenesis in the brain surrounding the glioma (Kleihues et al. 1997). The annual incidence of malignant gliomas is around .005% of the population. Therapy of malignant gliomas has not significantly changed in the past 20 years and currently includes tumor debulking, postoperative radiotherapy, and chemotherapy (Sasaki and Plate 1998). Of these, only radiotherapy has had a significant effect on patient survival. At present, the median survival time for glioblastoma patients is around 9 months following diagnosis.

One potential alternative therapy for the treatment of solid tumors is anti-angiogenesis. Folkman has proposed that the growth of solid tumors is angiogenesis-dependent (Gimbrone et al. 1972). In many human neoplasms, tumor formation is preceeded by an avascular phase. Tumor cell populations exceeding a few millimeters in size need a vascular network for further expansion. In this sense, absence of angiogenic activity can be considered rate-limiting for tumor growth (Folkman 1990). This hypothesis is supported by several animal models (reviewed in Folkman and Hanahan 1991; Hanahan and Folkman 1996). There is, therefore, considerable interest in evaluating whether specific inhibition of the vascularization of malignant tumors in animal models, and eventually in humans, will lead to tumor growth inhibition (Plate 1996).

3.3.1 Evidence that VEGF is a Tumor Angiogenesis Factor

VEGF is a secreted endothelial cell-specific growth factor (Leung et al. 1989) which induces angiogenesis and vascular permeability in vivo (Conolly et al. 1989; Keck et al. 1989; Roberts and Palade 1997) and acts as a survival factor for endothelial cells (Alon et al. 1995; Benjamin and Keshet 1997). In many tumor types, the expression of VEGF correlates with the degree of malignancy. VEGF is highly expressed in malignant gliomas, but to a much lesser extent in low-grade gliomas (Plate et al. 1992; for review see Plate and Risau 1995). VEGF expression is even lower in the normal adult brain (Plate et al. 1992). Intracellular oxygen tension is a major regulator of VEGF expression . In vitro, VEGF is hypoxia-inducible in glioma in cells (Shweiki et al. 1992) and in vivo is upregulated in palisading cells immediately adjacent to necroses (Shweiki et al. 1992; Plate et al. 1992). In vitro assays have shown that hypoxia increases both VEGF transcription and mRNA stability (Ikeda et al. 1995; Levy et al. 1996). Xenograft experiments using glioma cells stably transfected with a reporter gene under control of hypoxia-responsive elements of the VEGF gene suggest that hypoxia is the major force behind in vivo VEGF upregulation in perinecrotic palisading cells in gliomas (Damert et al. 1997).

The receptors for VEGF, VEGF-R1 (De Vries et al. 1992) and VEGF-R2 (Terman et al. 1992; Millauer et al. 1993) are expressed on proliferating and migrating endothelial cells during physiological angiogenesis in the developing embryo. VEGF receptors cannot be detected in normal adult brain, with the exception of plexus choroideus endothelium (Millauer et al. 1993; Breier et al. 1995; Dumont et al. 1995). Both receptors, however, are upregulated in tumor endothelial cells. VEGF-R1 and -R2 are expressed in tumor endothelial cells in malignant gliomas, whereas in lowgrade gliomas only VEGF-R1 expression could be detected, consistent with tumor-progression-associated receptor upregulation (Plate et al. 1994b; Hatva et al. 1995). Recent studies using cerebral slice cultures and cultured endothelial cells suggest that a hypoxia-inducible protein secreted by tumor cells induces VEGF receptor upregulation and that this factor is VEGF itself (Kremer et al. 1997; Barleon et al. 1997). Thus, VEGF induced by hypoxia may initiate the angiogenic cascade in a malignant tumor by induction of its receptors in endothelial cells, providing an auto-enhancing mechanism of tumor angiogenesis (Kremer et al. 1997). These observations and the finding that VEGF protein is detected predominantly around the vascular target cells suggest that VEGF acts as a paracrine growth factor in situ (Plate et al. 1992). In addition, these observations suggest that the VEGF/VEGF receptor system could be a promising target for anti-angiogenic therapy in malignant brain tumors (Plate 1996; Stratmann et al. 1997).

3.3.2 Tie2 and Angiopoietins May Be Involved in Vascular Remodeling

The recruitment of perivascular support cells (smooth muscle cells and pericytes) is a prominent feature of glioblastoma blood vessels (Kleihues et al. 1997). The presence of microvascular proliferations is considered a diagnostic feature of malignant gliomas by the World Health Organization (WHO 1993). It has been shown that the majority of cells of glioblastoma blood vessels are of pericyte or smooth muscle cell origin (Haddah et al. 1992; Wesseling et al. 1995). Although the relevance of this finding for tumor vascular biology is unclear, recent results suggest that in glioblastomas pericyte recruitment is regulated by the PDGF/PDGF receptor system and that the tie2/angiopoietin system is also involved. Thus, whereas in normal, mature blood vessels Ang-1 expression exceeds Ang-2 expression, the opposite is true for tumor blood vessels (Stratmann et al. 1998). Thus, Ang-2 upregulation appears to be a prerequisite for the induction of tumor angiogenesis. These observations are in line with the proposed role of angiopoietin-2 in destabilizing the vessel wall (Hanahan 1997). A role for tie2 in breast cancer angiogenesis has recently been proposed (Lin et al. 1997). Further in vivo experiments are needed to clarify the putative roles of tie2 and angiopoietins in glioma angiogenesis.

3.3.3 Inhibition of the VEGF/VEGF Receptor System in Experimental Tumors

Several approaches have been used for targeting the VEGF/VEGF receptor system (Table 2). These include (a) application of monoclonal anti-VEGF antibodies, (b) injection of retroviruses encoding dominant-negative-acting VEGF receptor mutants, (c) injection of soluble VEGF receptor extracellular domains, (d) application of low molecular weight VEGF receptor inhibitors, VEGF-specific ribozymes, and anti-VEGF-R2 antibodies, and (e) expression of antisense VEGF constructs in tumor cells (Saleh et al. 1996; Cheng et al. 1996; Claffey et al. 1996). Briefly, all approaches have proven successful in in vivo test systems, because tumor angiogenesis was inhibited and tumor growth was slowed down. Furthermore, in rats treated with a dominant-negative-acting VEGF-R2, a two- to fourfold increase in survival time was observed (Millauer et al. 1996 and unpublished results). Systemic treatment of rats with intracranial GS9L gliomas with a synthetic VEGF-R2 inhibitor also leads to a significant increase in survival time (our own unpublished

Table 2. Current strategies to target the VEGF/VEGF receptor system in tumor therapy

Approach	References
Anti-VEGF antibodies	Kim et al. 1993; Kondo et al. 1993
VEGF-specific ribozymes	Ke et al. 1998
Antisense VEGF	Saleh et al. 1996; Cheng et al. 1996; Claffey et al. 1996
VEGF antagonists	Siemeister et al. 1998
Soluble VEGF-R1	Kendall and Thomas 1993
Soluble VEGF-R2	Lin et al. 1998
Dominant-negative VEGF-R2	Millauer et al. 1994, 1996; Stratmann et al. 1997
Low molecular weight inhibitor of VEGF-R2	Strawn et al. 1996
Anti-VEGF-R2 antibodies	Skobe et al. 1997

results). Taken together, these results demonstrate an important role of the VEGF/VEGF receptor system in regulating brain tumor angiogenesis in animal models. Several of the above mentioned experimental approaches are currently being tested by various groups for their suitability in human tumor therapy.

3.4 Cerebral Ischemia

Several reports indicate that VEGF and its receptors can be upregulated in adult tissues under pathological conditions associated with tissue hypoxia/ischemia. Angiogenesis has, for example, been described to occur after cerebrovascular hypoxia and ischemia (Krupinski et al. 1994). The induction of angiogenesis in these cases can be interpreted as a natural defense mechanism in which the expression of VEGF leads to increased vascularization and enhanced partial oxygen pressure in the respective tissue. Upregulation of VEGF and its receptors has been described in rodent models of focal cerebral ischemia (Kovácz et al. 1996; Hayashi et al. 1997; Lennmyr et al. 1998) and chronic normobaric hypoxia (Ment et al. 1997; Patt et al. 1998). We observed cell-type-specific upregulation of VEGF mRNA in the peri-ischemic area in rats subjected to permanent, middle cerebral artery occlusion (MCAO). VEGF mRNA was upregulated beginning 3 h after the onset of MCAO and was present 7 days afterward (our own unpublished observations). Furthermore, we observed a three- to fourfold increase in vascular density, as well as depression of apoptosis in the peri-ischemic area, suggesting a functional response of the injured brain to VEGF secretion.

3.5 Clinical Application of Angiogenesis Research: Anti-angiogenesis and Therapeutic Angiogenesis

In principle, both inhibition and stimulation of angiogenesis appear to be suitable therapeutic goals, depending on the underlying disease. For malignant tumors such as glioblastoma, anti-angiogenesis has received considerable attention. In contrast, cerebrovascular ischemia may be particularly well-suited for therapeutic angiogenesis because most other methods have failed in the treatment of brain infarction.

Anti-angiogenic tumor therapy appears suitable for highly vascularized tumors in which no sure therapy is available. This holds true for most carcinomas, sarcomas, and malignant gliomas. Several compounds with anti-angiogenic effects are presently undergoing phase I/II clinical trials. At present, it is difficult to predict which approach or combination of approaches will be most suitable for anti-angiogenic tumor therapy in humans. Although many reports convincingly stress the importance of the VEGF/VEGF receptor system for tumor angiogenesis, other growth factor receptor systems, including angiopoietins and TIE receptor tyrosine kinases (Hatva et al. 1995; Lin et al. 1997; Stratmann et al. 1998), may be involved. It will be important to determine whether different tumor types take advantage of different angiogenic pathways. If so, certain tumors would require individual anti-angiogenic approaches. Another important question is whether tumor cells have the ability to switch from one angiogenic pathway to another in order to satisfy their need for oxygen and nutritients. This would imply the necessity to block several putative angiogenesis pathways in a single tumor.

Therapeutic angiogenesis may be attractive for ischemic cerebrovascular disease. The potential of VEGF to induce angiogenesis in vivo has been proven in several model systems (Drake and Little 1995; Flamme et al. 1995; Mühlhauser et al. 1995; Feucht et al. 1997; Rosenstein et al. 1998). Exogenous VEGF application has been tested in several model systems, including hind limb (Takeshita et al. 1994) and myocardial ischemia (Banai et al. 1994), and is currently in clinical use on patients with peripheral artery disease (Isner et al. 1996a, b). Our study of angiogenesis and VEGF expression in focal cerebral rat ischemia, as well as the study by Hayashi et al. (1998) using recombinant VEGF in a ceberal ischemia model, may provide the experimental basis for treating ischemic cerebrovascular disease by VEGF or VEGF analogues.

Acknowledgements. Due to space limitations, only part of the relevant literature could be mentioned here. The work described in this manuscript represents a long-standing, ongoing collaboration with Dr. Werner Risau, Bad Nauheim, Germany, and was supported by grants from the Deutsche Krebshilfe, the German Bundesministerium für Bildung und Forschung, the Deutsche Forschungsgemeinschaft, the Max Planck Society, and the Center for Clinical Research I of the Freiburg University Medical School.

References

Alon T, Hemo I, Itin A, Peér J, Stone J, Keshet E (1995) Vascular endothelial growth factor acts as a survival factor for newly formed retinal vessels and has implications for retinopathy of prematurity. Nat Med 1:1024–1028

Banai S, Jaklitsch MT, Shou M, Lazarous DF, Scheinowitz M, Bito M, Biro S, Epstein SE, Unger EF (1994) Angiogenic-induced enhancement of collateral blood flow to ischemic myocardium by vascular endothelial growth factor in dogs. Circulation 89:2183–2198

Barleon B, Siemeister G, Martiny-Baron G, Weindel K, Herzog C, Marmé D (1997) Vascular endothelial growth factor up-regulates ist receptor fms-like tyrosine kinase 1 (flt-1) and a soluble variant of flt-1 in human vascular endothelial cells. Cancer Res 57:5421–5425

Benjamin LE, Keshet E (1997) Conditional switching of vascular endothelial growth factor (VEGF) expression in tumors: induction of endothelial cell shedding and regression of hemangioblastoma-like vessels by VEGF withdrawal. Proc Natl Acad Sci USA 94:8761–8766

Breier G, Damert A, Plate KH, Risau W (1992) Angiogenesis in embryos and ischemic diseases. Thromb Haemost 78:678–683

Breier G, Clauss M, Risau W (1995) Coordinate expression of vascular endothelial growth factor receptor-1 (flt-1) and its ligand suggests a paracrine regulation of murine vascular development. Dev Dyn 204:228–239

Carmeliet P, Ferreira V, Breier G, Pollefeyt S, Kieckens L, Gertsenstein M, Fahrig M, Vandenhoec A, Harpal K, Eberhard C, Desclerc C, Pawling M, Moons L, Collen D, Risau W, Nagy A (1996) Abnormal blood vessel development and lethality in embryos lacking a single VEGF allele. Nature 380:435–439

Cheng SY, Huang HJS, Nagane M, Ji XD, Wang DG, Shih CCY, Arap W, Huang CM, Cavenee WK (1996) Suppression of glioblastoma angiogenicity and tumourigenicity by inhibition of endogenous expression of vascular endothelial growth factor. Proc Natl Acad Sci USA 93:8502–8507

Claffey KP, Brown LF, Delaguila LF, Tognazzi K, Yeo KT, Manseau EJ, Dvorak HF (1996) Expression of vascular permeability factor vascular endothelial growth factor by melanoma cells increases tumour growth, angiogenesis, and experimental metastasis. Cancer Res 56:172–181

Conolly DT, Heuvelman DM, Nelson R, Olander JV, Eppley BL, Delfino JJ, Siegel NR, Leimgruber RM, Feder J (1989) Tumor vascular permeability factor stimulates endothelial cell growth and angiogenesis. J Clin Invest 84:1470–1478

Damert A, Machein M, Breier G, Fujita MQ, Hanahan D, Risau W, Plate KH (1997) Up-regulation of vascular endothelial growth factor expression in a rat glioma is conferred by two distinct hypoxia-driven mechanisms. Cancer Res 57:3860–3864

Davis S, Aldrich TH, Jones PF, Acheson A, Compton DL, Jain V, Ryan TE, Bruno J, Radziejewski C, Maisonpierre PC, Yancopoulos GD (1996) Isolation of angiopoietin-1, a ligand for the tie2 receptor, by secretion-trap expression cloning. Cell 87:1161–1169

De Vries C, Escobedo JA, Ueno H, Houck K, Ferrara N, Williams LT (1992) The fms-like tyrosine kinase, a receptor for vascular endothelial growth factor. Science 255:989–991

Drake CJ, Little CD (1995) Exogenous vascular endothelial growth factor induces malformed and hyperfused vessels during embryonic neovascularization. Proc Natl Acad Sci USA 92:7657–7661

Dumont DJ, Yamaguchi TP, Conlon RA, Rossant J, Breitman ML (1992) Tek, novel tyrosine kinase gene located on mouse chromosome 4, is expressed in endothelial cells and their presumptive precursors. Oncogene 7:1471–1480

Dumont DJ, Gradwohl G, Fong G-H, Puri MC, Gertsenstein M, Auerbach A, Breitman ML (1994) Dominant-negative and targeted null mutations in the endothelial receptor tyrosine kinase, tek, reveal a critical role in vasculogenesis of the embryo. Genes Dev 8:1897–1909

Dumont D, Fong G-H, Puir MC, Gradwohl G, Alitalo K, Breitman M (1995) Vascularization of the mouse embryo: a study of flk-1, tek, tie, and vascular endothelial growth factor expression during development. Dev Dyn 203:80–92

Ferrara N, Carver-Moore K, Chen H, Dowd M, Lu L, O´Shea KS, Powell-Braxton L, Hillan K, Moore MW (1996) Heterozygous embryonic lethality induced by targeted inactivation of the VEGF gene. Nature 380:439–442

Feucht M, Christ B, Wilting J (1997) VEGF induces cardiovascular malformation and embryonic lethality. Am J Pathol 151:1407–1416

Flamme I, von Reuterrn M, Drexler HCA, Syed-Ali S, Risau W (1995) Overexpression of vascular endothelial growth factor in the avian embryo induces hypervascularization and increases vascular permeability without alterations of embryonic pattern formation. Dev Biol 171:399–4141

Folkman J (1990) What is the evidence that tumors are angiogenesis dependent? J Natl Cancer Inst 82:4–6

Folkman J, Hanahan D (1991) Expression of the angiogenic phenotype during development of murine and human cancer. In: Brugge J (ed) Origins of human cancer: a comprehensive review. Cold Spring Harbor Laboratory Press, Cold Spring Harbor, pp 803–814

Fong G-H, Rossant J, Gertsenstein M, Breitman ML (1995) Role of the flt-1 receptor tyrosine kinase in regulating the assembly of vascular endothelium. Nature 376:66–70

Gimbrone MA Jr, Leapman SB, Cotran RS, Folkman J (1972) Tumor dormancy in vivo by prevention of neovascularization. J Exp Med 136:261–276

Haddah SF, Moore SA, Schelper RL, Goeken JA (1992) Vascular smooth muscle hyperplasia underlies the formation of glomeruloid vascular structures of glioblastoma multiforme. J Neuropathol Exp Neurol 51:488–492

Hanahan D (1997) Signaling vascular morphogenesis and maintenance. Science 277:48–50

Hanahan D, Folkman J (1996) Patterns and emerging mechanisms of the angiogenic switch during tumorigenesis. Cell 86:353–364

Hatva E, Kaipainen A, Jääskelainen J, Paetau A, Haltia M, Alitalo K (1995) Expression of endothelial cell-specific receptor tyrosine kinases and growth factors in human brain tumours. Am J Pathol 146:368–378

Hayashi T, Abe K, Suzuki H, Itoyama Y (1997) Rapid induction of vascular endothelial growth factor gene expression after transient middle cerebral artery occlusion in rats. Stroke 28:2039–2044

Hayashi T, Abe K, Itoyama Y (1998) Reduction of ischemic damage by application of vascular endothelial growth factor in rat brain after transient ischemia. J Cereb Blood Flow Metab 18:887–895

Ikeda E, Achen MG, Breier G, Risau W (1995) Hypoxia-induced transcriptional activation and increased mRNA stability of vascular endothelial growth factor in C6 glioma cells. J Biol Chem 270:19761–19766

Isner JM, Pieczek A, Schainfield R, Blair R, Haley L, Asahara T, Rosenfield K, Razvi S, Walsh K, Symes JF (1996a) Clinical evidence of angiogenesis after arterial gene transfer of phVEGF165 in patient with ischaemic limb. Lancet 348:370–374

Isner JM, Walsh K, Symes J, Pieczek A, Takeshita S, Lowry J, Rosenfield K, Weir L, Brogi E, Jurayi D (1996b) Arterial gene transfer for therapeutic angiogenesis in patients with peripheral artery disease. Hum Gen Ther 7:959–988

Ke LD, Fueyo J, Chen X, Steck PA, Shi YX, Im SA, Yung WKA (1998) A novel approach to glioma gene therapy: down-regulation of the vascular endothelial growth factor in glioma cells using ribozymes. Int J Cancer 12:1391–1396

Keck PJ, Hauser S, Krivi G, Sanzo K, Warren T, Feder J, Conolly DT (1989) Vascular permeability factor, an endothelial cell mitogen related to PDGF. Science 246:1309–1312

Kendall RL, Thomas KA (1993) Inhibition of vascular endothelial growth factor activity by an endogenously encoded soluble receptor. Proc Natl Acad Sci USA 90:10705–10709

Kim JB, Li B, Winer J, Armanini M, Gillett N, Phillips HS, Ferrara N (1993) Inhibition of vascular endothelial growth factor-induced angiogenesis suppresses tumour growth in vivo. Nature 362:841–844

Kleihues P, Burger PC, Plate KH, Ohgaki H, Cavenee WK (1997) Glioblastoma. In: Kleihues P, Cavenee WK (eds) Pathology and genetics of tumours of the nervous system. International Agency for Research on Cancer, Lyon, pp 16–24

Kondo S, Asano M, Suzuki H (1993) Significance of vascular endothelial growth factor / vascular permeability factor for solid tumor growth, and its inhibition by the antibody. Biochem Biophys Res Commun 194:1234–1241

Kovácz Z, Ikezaki K, Samoto K, Inamura T, Fukui M (1996) VEGF and flt: expression time kinetics in rat brain infarct. Stroke 27:1865–1873

Kremer C, Breier G, Risau W, Plate KH (1997) Upregulation of flk-1/VEGF receptor-2 by its ligand in a cerebral slice culture system. Cancer Res 57:3852–3859

Krupinski J, Kaluza J, Kumar P, Kumar S, Wang JM (1994) Role of angiogenesis in patients with cerebral ischemic stroke. Stroke 25:1794–1798

Lennmyr F, Ata KA, Funa K, Olsson Y, Terént A (1998) Expression of vascular endothelial growth factor (VEGF) and its receptors (Flt-1 and Flk-1) following permanent and transient occlusion of the middle cerebral artery in the rat. J Neuropathol Exp Neurol 57:874–882

Leung DW, Cachianes G, Kuang W-J, Goeddel DV, Ferrara N (1989) Vascular endothelial growth factor is a secreted angiogenic mitogen. Science 246:1306–1309

Levy AP, Levy NS, Goldberg MA (1996) Post-transcriptional regulation of vascular endothelial growth factor by hypoxia. J Biol Chem 271:2746–2753

Lin P, Polverini P, Dewhirst M, Shan S, Rao PS, Peters K (1997) Inhibition of tumor angiogenesis using a soluble receptor establishes a role for Tie2 in pathologic vascular growth. J Clin Invest 100:2072–2078

Lin P, Sankar S, Shan S, Dewhirst MW, Polverini PJ, Quinn TQ, Peters KG (1998) Inhibition of tumor growth by targeting tumor endothelium using a soluble vascular endothelial growth factor receptor. Cell Growth Differ 9:49–58

Maisonpierre PC, Goldfarb M, Yancopoulos GD, Gao G (1993) Distinct rat genes with related profiles of expression define a TIE receptor tyrosine kinase family. Oncogene 8:1631–1637

Maisonpierre PC, Suri C, Jones PF, Bartunkova S, Wiegand SJ, Radziejewski C, Compton D, McClain J, Aldrich T, Papadopoulos N, Daly TJ, Davis S, Sato TN, Yancopoulos GD (1997) Angiopoietin-2, a natural antagonist for tie2 that disrupts in vivo angiogenesis. Science 277:55–60

Ment LR, Stewart WB, Fronc R, Seashore C, Mahooti S, Scaramuzzino D, Madri JA (1997) Vascular endothelial growth factor mediates reactive angiogenesis in the postnatal developung brain. Brain Res Dev Brain Res 100:52–61

Millauer B, Wizigmann-Voos S, Schnürch H, Martinez R, Moller NPH, Risau W, Ullrich A (1993) High affinity VEGF binding and developmental expression suggests flk-1 as a major regulator of vasculogenesis and angiogenesis. Cell 72:835–846

Millauer B, Shawver L, Plate KH, Risau W, Ullrich A (1994) Glioblastoma growth inhibited in vivo by a dominant-negative Flk-1 mutant. Nature 367:576–578

Millauer B, Longhi MP, Plate KH, Shawver LK, Risau W, Ullrich A, Strawn LM (1996) Dominant-negative inhibition of flk-1 suppresses the growth of many tumour types in vivo. Cancer Res 56:1615–1620

Moses MA, Langer R (1991) Inhibitors of angiogenesis. Biotechnology 9:630–634

Mühlhauser J, Merill MJ, Pili R, Maeda H, Bacic M, Bewig B, Passaniti A, Edwards NA, Crystal RG, Capogrossi MC (1995) VEGF165 expressed by a replication-deficient recombinant adenovirus vector induces angiogenesis in vivo. Circ Res 77:1077–1086

Patt S, Danner S, Hottenrott G, Théallier-Jankó A, Breier G, Plate KH, Cervós-Navarro J (1998) Upregulation of vascular endothelial growth factor in severe chronic brain hypoxia of the rat. Neurosci Lett 252:199–202

Plate KH (1996) Gene therapy of malignant glioma via inhibition of tumor angiogenesis. Cancer Metast Rev 15:237–240

Plate KH, Risau W (1995) Angiogenesis in malignant gliomas. Glia 15:339–347

Plate KH, Breier G, Weich HA, Risau W (1992) Vascular endothelial growth factor is a potential tumour angiogenesis factor in human gliomas in vivo. Nature 359:845–848

Plate KH, Breier G, Risau W (1994a) Molecular mechanisms of developmental and tumour angiogenesis. Brain Pathol 4:207–218

Plate KH, Breier G, Weich HA, Mennel HD, Risau W (1994b) Vascular endothelial growth factor and glioma angiogenesis: coordinate induction of VEGF receptors, distribution of VEGF protein and possible in vivo regulatory mechanisms. Int J Cancer 59:520–529

Puri MC, Rossant J, Alitalo K, Bernstein A, Partanen J (1995) The receptor tyrosine kinase TIE is required for integrity and survival of vascular endothelial cells. EMBO J 14:5884–5891

Risau W (1995) Differentiation of endothelium. FASEB J 9:926–933

Risau W (1997) Mechanisms of angiogenesis. Nature 386:671–674

Roberts WG, Palade GE (1997) Neovasculature induced by vascular endothelial growth factor is fenestrated. Cancer Res 57:765–772

Rosenstein JM, Mani N, Silvermann WF, Krum JM (1998) Patterns of brain angiogenesis after vascular endothelial growth factor administration in vitro and in vivo. Proc Natl Acad Sci USA 95:7086–7091

Saleh M, Stacker SA, Wilks AF (1996) Inhibition of growth of C6 glioma cells in vivo by expression of antisense vascular endothelial growth factor sequence. Cancer Res 56:393–401

Sasaki M, Plate KH (1998) Gene therapy of malignant gliomas: recent advances in experimental and clinical studies. Ann Oncol 9:1155–1166

Sato TN, Tozawa Y, Deutsch U, Wolburg-Buchholz K, Fujiwara Y, Gendron-Maguire M, Gridley T, Wolburg H, Risau W, Quin Y (1995) Distinct roles of the receptor tyrosine kinases tie-1 and tie-2 in blood vessel formation. Nature 376:70–74

Schnürch H, Risau W (1993) Expression of tie-2, a member of a novel family of receptor tyrosine kinases, in the endothelial lineage. Development 119:957–968

Shalaby F, Rossant J, Yamaguchi TP, Gertsenstein M, Wu X-F, Breitman ML, Schuh AC (1995) Failure of blood-island formation and vasculogenesis in flk-1 deficient mice. Nature 376:62–66

Shweiki D, Itin A, Soffer D, Keshet E (1992) Vascular endothelial growth factor induced by hypoxia may mediate hypoxia-initiated angiogenesis. Nature 359:843–845

Siemeister G, Schirner M, Reusch P, Barleon B, Marmé D, Martiny-Baron G (1998) An antagonistic vascular endothelial growth factor (VEGF) variant inhibits VEGF-stimulated receptor autophosphorylation and proliferation of human endothelial cells. PNAS 95:4625–4629

Skobe M, Rockwell P, Goldstein N, Vosseler S, Fusenig NE (1997) Halting angiogenesis suppresses carcinoma cell invasion. Nat Med 3:1222–1227

Stratmann A, Machein MR, Plate KH (1997) Anti-angiogenic gene therapy of malignant gliomas. Acta Neurochir (Wien) 68:105–110

Stratmann A, Risau W, Plate KH (1998) Cell-type specific expression of Angiopoietin-1 and Angiopoietin-2 suggest a role in glioblastoma angiogenesis. Am J Pathol 153:1459–1466

Strawn LM, McMahon G, App H, Schreck R, Kuchler WR, Longhi MP, Hui TH, Tang C, Levitzki A, Gazit A, Chen I, Keri G, Orfi L, Risau W, Flamme I, Ullrich A, Hirth KP, Shawver LK (1996) Flk-1 as a target for tumour growth inhibition. Cancer Res 56:3540–3545

Suri C, Jones PF, Patan S, Bartunkova S, Maisonpierre PC, Davis S, Sato N, Yancopoulos G (1996) Requisite role of angiopoietin-1, a ligand for the tie2 receptor, during embryonic angiogenesis. Cell 87:1171–1180

Takeshita S, Zheng LP, Brogi E, Kearney M, Pu L-Q, Bunting S. Ferrara N, Symes JF, Isner JM (1994) Therapeutic angiogenesis. J Clin Invest 93:662–670

Terman BC, Dougher-Vermazen M, Carrion ME, Dimitrov D, Armellino DC, Gospodarowicz D, Böhlen P (1992) Identification of the KDR tyrosine kinase as a receptor for vascular endothelial growth factor. Biochem Biophys Res Commun 187:1579–1586

Wesseling P, Schlingenmann RO, Rietveld FJR, Link M, Burger PC, Ruiter DJ (1995) Early and extensive contribution of pericytes/vascular smooth muscle cells to microvascular proliferation in glioblastoma multiforme – an immuno-light and immuno-electron microscopic study. J Neuropathol Exp Neurol 54:304–310

World Health Organization (1993) Kleihues P, Burger PC, Scheithauer BW (eds) Histological typing of tumours of the central nervous system. Springer, Berlin Heidelberg New York

4 TIE Receptors and Angiopoietins: Novel Modulators of Angiogenesis

T.N. Sato

4.1 Introduction

"Angiogenesis" has perhaps become as popular a word as "Michael Jordan", "Mickey Mouse", or "Titanic" over the last few years. A Medline reference search shows an exponential increase of the publications in the field of angiogenesis: in 1970, a search using "angiogenesis" as a key word identified only one paper published. Similar searches identified 38 publications in 1980, 198 in 1990, and 839 in 1997. This clearly indicates the recognition of the field of angiogenesis as one of the most important biomedical fields.

Angiogenesis is a process by which new vasculature forms during development and under disease conditions. It is now agreed that many human diseases, from cancer to aging, can benefit from therapeutical approaches for either inducing or inhibiting angiogenesis, depending on disease conditions. Despite the known therapeutical benefits, we are still in the early stages of understanding the basic cellular and molecular mechanisms underlying angiogenesis. In the following chapters, I will summarize the function and regulation of this novel receptor-ligand system in the vascular system, as well as its clinical relevance. In conclusion, I will also present my view of the potentially most exciting future areas of study in this field.

4.2 Receptor Tyrosine Kinases in Angiogenesis

One of the breakthroughs explaining how angiogenesis may be regulated at the molecular level came through the discovery of two novel classes of receptor tyrosine kinases expressed primarily in vascular endothelial cells. These are now called vascular endothelial growth factor (VEGF) receptors and tyrosine kinase with immunoglobulin domains and EGF repeat (TIE) receptors. VEGF receptors belong to one of the subclasses of the PDGF receptor family. Extracellular portion of all of the VEGF receptors consists of seven immunoglobulin-like domains. Currently there exist three known VEGF receptors, VEGF-R1, VEGF-R2, and VEGF-R3 (De Vries et al. 1992; Kaipainen et al. 1995; Millauer et al. 1993; Quinn et al. 1993). Their activities are regulated by at least four specific ligands, VEGF-A, VEGF-B, VEGF-C, and VEGF-D (Joukov et al. 1996; Mustonen and Alitalo 1995). This receptor-ligand system primarily regulates proliferation, survival, and/or permeability of vascular endothelial cells (Fong et al. 1995, 1996; Shalaby et al. 1995, 1997).

The other class of endothelial receptor tyrosine kinases is formed by TIE receptors, distinguished by their molecules' unique extracellular portion consisting of two immunoglobulin-like domains flanking three repeats of EGF-like domains and followed by three fibronectin type III repeats. Two TIE receptors, TIE1 (aka TIE) and TIE2 (aka TEK), are currently identified (Dumont et al. 1993; Iwama et al. 1993; Maisonpierre et al. 1993; Sato et al. 1993; Schnurch and Risau 1993). Two specific ligandsfor the TIE2 receptor have been identified, angiopoietin-1 and angiopoietin-2 (Davis et al. 1996; Maisonpierre et al. 1997; Suri et al. 1996).

4.3 TIE receptors

Both TIE1 and TIE2 were identified initially as novel receptor tyrosine kinases that are specifically expressed in vascular endothelial cells (Dumont et al. 1993; Iwama et al. 1993; Korhonen et al. 1992; Maisonpierre et al. 1993; Sato et al. 1993; Schnurch and Risau 1993). Their unique extracellular domain composition implicated the existence of unique ligands that may regulate the novel aspects of blood vessel formation in development and/or diseases. In situ hybridization of embryos and adult tissues clearly indicated the vascular endothelial cells as primary cells expressing both of these receptors. The first important implication of these receptors was made clear by analyses of TIE1 and TIE2 knockout mice (Dumont et al. 1994; Puri et al. 1995; Sato et al. 1995). This study showed TIE1 knockout mouse embryos dying between the midgestation and neonatal stages with severe edema and hemorrhage. This indicated that the TIE1 receptor is important for maintaining and/or developing vascular integrity, and perhaps survival of endothelial cells. TIE2 knockout mouse embryos died earlier, at the E9.5 stage, with malformation of the embryonic vascular network, suggesting the importance of the TIE2 receptor in vascular network remodeling. However, the detailed cellular and developmental processes regulated by TIE1 and TIE2 receptors still remain unclear.

4.4 Angiopoietins

The next breakthrough in understanding the mechanisms by which TIE receptors regulate blood vessel formation came from the discovery of specific ligands for the TIE2 receptor. Two specific ligands, angiopoietin-1 and angiopoietin-2, have been so far reported (Davis et al. 1996; Maisonpierre et al. 1997; Suri et al. 1996). Both of these angiopoietins belong to a novel class of secreted glycoproteins. They share two prominent domains, the coiled-coil domain followed by a fibrinogen-like domain. In cell culture systems, angiopoietin-1 was shown to bind specifically to the TIE2 receptor and, upon binding, to induce autophosphorylation of cytoplasmic tyrosine residue(s) of the receptor, a hallmark of its activation. Furthermore, angiopoietin-1 knockout mouse embryos exhibit a specific vascular phenotype similar to that of TIE2 knockout embryos. These in vitro biochemical and in vivo genetic analyses confirmed that angiopoietin-1 is a specific activating ligand for the TIE2 receptor. In contrast, angiopoietin-2 binds to the TIE2 receptor but fails to activate the TIE2 receptor expressed on the surface of cultured endothelial cells. In the presence of both angiopoietin-1 and angiopoietin-2 in culture media, angiopoietin-2 inhibits TIE2 receptor activation mediated by angiopoietin-1. Furthermore, misexpression of angiopoietin-2 in embryonic vasculature resulted in vascular malformation as observed in both angiopoietin-1 and TIE2 receptor knockout mouse embryos. These in vitro and in vivo studies suggest that angiopoietin-2 is an endogenous antagonist for the TIE2 receptor. Expression of both angiopoietin-1 and -2 was detected predominantly in nonendothelial cells immediately adjacent to vascular endothelial cells such as smooth muscle and mesenchymal cells. This pattern of expression suggests the paracrine mechanism of the TIE2 receptor function by angiopoietins (Folkman and D'Amore 1996). Furthermore, the existence of an endogenous agonist and antagonist for the TIE2 receptor suggests complex positive and negative regulations of blood vessel formation by this ligand-receptor system (Hanahan 1997).

With the discovery of angiopoietins as specific ligands for the TIE2 receptor, downstream signaling mechanisms of the TIE2 receptor are now beginning to be revealed. Furthermore, it has now become feasible to develop more sophisticated in vitro assay systems for studying how angiopoietins regulate the cellular behavior of endothelial cells.

4.5 TIE Receptors and Angiopoietins in Human Diseases

As we understand more about the basic mechanisms of vascular development regulated by angiopoietin-TIE2 receptor system, we have also begun to learn about the role of this ligand-receptor system in human diseases as well.

4.5.1 Venous Malformation Diseases

Recently one form of human venous malformation disease was shown to be caused by the single amino acid substitution mutation of the cytoplasmic region of the TIE2 receptor (Vikkula et al. 1996). This malformation results from the defective interaction between endothelial cells and smooth muscle cells. Therefore, it is possible that the angiopoietin-TIE2 system may be involved in this paracrine cell-cell interaction, an important process underlying vascular network remodeling.

4.5.2 Tumor Angiogenesis

The TIE2 receptor has been shown to be expressed in endothelial cells of blood vessels in tumors and, most recently, inhibition of the TIE2 receptor activity in a few animal models resulted in significant inhibition of angiogenesis and subsequent shrinkage of tumors (Lin et al. 1997, 1998; Peters et al. 1998). This clearly indicates the important role of the TIE2 receptor in tumor angiogenesis.

4.5.3 Other Diseases

Based on the clear implications of the important roles of TIE receptors and angiopoietins in developing embryonic vasculature, as well as the recent data in venous malformation disease and tumor angiogenesis described above, we will certainly begin to see more data (we hope, encouraging ones!) on the roles of angiopoietins and TIE receptors in other human diseases where blood vessel formation and regression play important roles, including ischemic heart and limb diseases, wound healing, AIDS, etc.

4.6 Future Developments

During the last five years since the discovery of TIE receptors, we gained a significant amount of knowledge of the biochemical properties and biological functions of the angiopoietin-TIE receptor system. There are also now a few encouraging results on the therapeutic use of this ligand-receptor system in various human diseases. The following is a list of what I consider the most promising research fields for new discoveries in the angiopoietin-TIE receptor field:

1. To define the signaling pathways mediated by the angiopoietin-TIE2 receptor, as well as the exact cellular processes regulated by this ligand-receptor pathway. We still do not know much about the mechanisms by which the angiopoietin-TIE2 receptor regulates blood vessel formation. Therefore, it would be essential to define the biochemical pathways and the endothelial cell behavior regulated by this ligand-receptor system.
2. Study of the interactions between angiopoietin-TIE2 receptor signaling and that of other ligand-receptor systems. All endothelial behavior is the result of integration of multiple signaling pathways. Therefore, it will be important to define how angiopoietin-TIE2 receptor signaling may interact with other signaling pathways regulated by other ligand-receptor systems, such as VEGF-VEGF-receptors.
3. Discovery of a ligand for the TIE1 receptor. Although we have learned quite a lot about the TIE2 receptor, due to the discovery of angiopoietins, a ligand for the TIE1 receptor is still unknown. Identification of such a ligand for this orphan receptor will certainly shed light on the function of this molecule.
4. The study of angiopoietin-TIE2 receptor functions in human disease and development of effective therapeutic reagents based on this ligand-receptor system.

Now that the TIE2 receptor has been clearly shown to be involved in some of the human diseases described above, it is encouraging to examine the roles of this ligand-receptor system in many other human diseases in which blood vessel formation and regression are assumed to shape their pathogenesis. These studies may eventually lead to the invention of novel and more effective therapies for many human diseases.

References

Davis S, Aldrich TH, Jones PF, Acheson A, Bruno J, Radjiewski C, Compton D, Maisonpierre PC, Yancopoulos GD (1996) Isolation of angiopoietin-1, a ligand for the TIE2 receptor, by secretion-trap expression cloning. Cell 87:1161–1169

De Vries C, Escobedo JA, Ueno H, Houck K, Ferrara N, Williams LT (1992) The fms-like tyrosine kinase, a receptor for vascular endothelial growth factor. Science 255:989–991

Dumont DJ, Gradwohl GJ, Fong G-H, Auerbach R, Breitman ML (1993) The endothelial-specific receptor tyrosine kinase, tek, is a member of a new subfamily of receptors. Oncogene 8:1293–1301

Dumont DJ, Gradwohl G, Fong G-H, Puri MC, Gerstenstein M, Auerbach A, Breitman ML (1994) Domintant-negative and targeted null mutations in the endothelial receptor tyrosine kinase, tek, reveal a critical role in vasculogenesis of the embryo. Genes Dev 8:1897–1909

Folkman J, D'Amore PA (1996) Blood vessel formation: what is its molecular basis? Cell 87:1153–1155

Fong G-H, Rossant J, Breitman ML (1995) Role of the Flt-1 receptor tyrosine kinase in regulationg the assembly of vascular endothelium. Nature 376:66–70

Fong G-H, Klingensmith J, Wood CR, Rossant J, Breitman ML (1996) Regulation of flt-1 expression during mouse embryogenesis suggests a role in the establishment of vascular endothelium. Dev Dyn 207:1–10

Hanahan D (1997) Signaling vascular morphogenesis and maintenance. Science 277:48–50

Iwama A, Hamaguchi I, Hashiyama M, Murayama Y, Yasunaga K, Suda T (1993) Molecular cloning and characterization of mouse Tie and Tek receptor tyrosine kinase genes and their expression in hematopoietic stem cells. Biochem Biophys Res Commun 195:301–309

Joukov V, Pajusola K, Kaipainen A, Chilov D, Lahtinen I, Kukk E, Saksela O, Kalkkinen N, Alitalo K(1996) A novel vascular endothelial growth factor, VEGF-C, is a ligand for the Flt4 (VEGFR-3) and KDR (VEGFR-2) receptor tyrosine kinases. EMBO J 15:290–298

Kaipainen A, Korhonen J, Mustonen T, van Hinsbergh VWM, Fang G-H, Dumont D, Breitman M, Alitalo K (1995) Expression of the fms-like tyrosine kinase 4 gene becomes restricted to lymphatic endothelium during development. Proc Natl Acad Sci USA 92:3566–3570

Korhonen J, Partanen J, Armstrong E, Vaahtokari A, Elenius K, Jalkanen M, Alitalo K (1992) Enhanced expression of the tie receptor tyrosine kinase in endlthelial cells during neovascularization. Blood 80:2548–2555

Lin P, Polverini P, Dewhirst M, Shan S, Rao PS, Peters K (1997) Inhibition of tumor angiogenesis using a soluble receptor establishes a role for Tie2 in pathologic vascular growth. J Clin Invest 100:2072–2078

Lin P, Buxton JA, Acheson A, Radziejewski C, Maisonpierre PC, Yancopoulos GD, Channon KM, Hale LP, Dewhirst MW, George SE, Peters KG (1998) Antiangiogenic gene therapy targeting the endothelium-specific receptor tyrosine kinase tie2. Proc Natl Acad Sci USA 95:8829–8834

Maisonpierre PC, Goldfarb M, Yancopoulos GD, Gao G (1993) Distinct rat genes with related profiles of expression define a TIE receptor tyrosine kinase family. Oncogene 8:1631–1637

Maisonpierre PC, Suri C, Jones PF, Bartunkova S, Wiegand SJ, Radziejewski C, Compton D, McClain J, Aldrich TH, Papadapoulos N, Daly TJ, Davis S, Sato TN, Yancopoulos GD (1997) Angiopoietin-2:a natural antagonist for Tie2 that disrupts in vivo angiogenesis. Science 277:55–60

Millauer B, Wizigmann VS, Schnurch H, Martinez R, Moller NP, Risau W, Ullrich A (1993) High affinity VEGF binding and developmental expression suggest Flk-1 as a major regulator of vasculogenesis and angiogenesis. Cell 72:835–846

Mustonen T, Alitalo K (1995) Endothelial receptor tyrosine kinases involved in angiogenesis. J Cell Biol 129:895–898

Peters KG, Coogan A, Berry D, Marks J, Iglehart JD, Kontos CD, Rao P, Sankar S, Trogan E (1998) Expression of Tie2/Tek in breast tumor vasculature provides a new marker for evaluation of tumour angiogenesis. Br J Cancer 77:51–56

Puri MC, Rossant J, Alitalo K, Bernstein A, Partanen J (1995) The receptor tyrosine kinase TIE is required for integrity and survival of vascular endothelial cells. EMBO J 14:5884–5891

Quinn TP, Peters KG, De VC, Ferrara N, Williams LT (1993) Fetal liver kinase 1 is a receptor for vascular endothelial growth factor and is selectively expressed in vascular endothelium. Proc Natl Acad Sci USA 90:7533–7537

Sato TN, Qin Y, Kozak CA, Audus KL (1993) tie-1 and tie-2 define another class of putative receptor tyrosine kinase genes expressed in early embryonic vascular system. Proc Natl Acad Sci USA 90:9355–9358

Sato TN, Tozawa Y, Deutsch U, Wolburg-Buchholz K, Fujiwara Y, Gendron-Maguire M, Gridley T, Wolburg H, Risau W, Qin Y (1995) Distinct roles of the receptor tyrosine kinases Tie-1 and Tie-2 in blood vessel formation. Nature 376:70–74

Schnurch H, Risau W (1993) Expression of tie-2, a member of a novel family of receptor tyrosine kinases, in the endothelial cell lineage. Development 119:957–968

Shalaby F, Rossant J, Yamaguchi TP, Breitman M, Schuh AC (1995) Failure of blood island formation, vasculogenesis, and hematopoiesis in flk-1 deficient mice. Nature 376:62–66

Shalaby F, Ho J, Stanford WL, Fischer K-D, Schuh AC, Schwartz L, Bernstein A, Rossant J (1997) A requirement for Flk1 in primitive and definitive hematopoiesis and vasculogenesis. Cell 89:981–990

Suri C, Jones PF, Patan S, Bartunkova S, Maisonpierre PC, Davis S, Sato TN, Yancopoulos GD (1996) Requisite role of angiopoietin-1, a ligand for the TIE2 receptor, during embryonic angiogenesis. Cell 87:1171–1180

Vikkula M, Boon LM, Carraway KL, Calvert JT, Diamonti AJ, Goumnerov B, Pasyk KA, Marchuk DA, Warman ML, Cantley LC, Mulliken JB, Olsen BR (1996) Vascular dysmorphogenesis caused by an activating mutation in the receptor tyrosine kinase TIE2. Cell 87:1181–1190

5 Collateral and Capillary Formation – A Comparison

E. Deindl, W. Schaper

5.1 Introduction

Vascular occlusive diseases are the major cause of mortality in Western civilization. The devastating consequences of ischemia and infarction could be prevented by the timely induction of collateral artery growth. Knowing the molecular mechanisms responsible for vessel growth is the basic requirement for the development of effective therapies.

In the postnatal organism, two types of vessel growth exist: angiogenesis, which is defined as the sprouting of capillaries, and arteriogenesis, the growth of collateral arteries from preexisting arteriolar connections. The mechanisms of angiogenesis have been studied intensively during the last 20 years. Results show that growth factors, potent regulators of cellular functions like proliferation and migration, play an important role in capillary sprouting. Clinical studies already showed evidence that vascular endothelial growth factor (VEGF) is a potent angiogenic factor in humans (Isner et al. 1996). However, to induce capillary sprouting does not solve the problem completely. Indeed, it ensures the supply of a tissue with metabolites and oxygen, but the preceding step is missing – the enhancement of collateral artery development, providing the important source of blood flow to the ischemic area. VEGF is only a mitogen for endothelial cells. True collateral artery growth, however, requires the proliferation of endothelial cells and smooth muscle cells. Up to now, little is known about the mechanisms of collateral artery growth. Previous studies showed that they grow from preexisting arteriolar connections (Schaper and Schaper 1993). Pressure gradients develop along the arterioles, leading to the generation of shear stress. In most models, arteriogenesis is temporally and spatially dissociated from ischemia (Schaper and Schaper 1993), in contrast to capillary sprouting, which is mainly observed in ischemic areas (Plate et al. 1992; Schaper and Schaper 1993; Folkman 1995; Görge et al. 1989).

5.2 The Animal Model

To analyze whether angiogenesis and arteriogenesis obey one and the same mechanism and to characterize the various mechanisms of arteriogenesis, we developed an in vivo model that can be functionally evaluated. Occlusion of the femoral artery of the rabbit results (in the absence of ischemia) in collateral growth in the upper leg (Fig. 1), and – due to ischemia – in capillary sprouting in the lower leg. The collateral arteries develop between branches of the arteria circumflexa femoris lateralis and the arteriae genualis, as well as between branches of the arteria femoralis profunda and the arteria saphena parva. The growth of true collateral arteries from preexisting arteriolar anastomoses begins as soon as 24 h after occlusion, with maximum proliferation during the first 3 days after occlusion. KI67 and BrdU staining revealed a massive proliferation of endothelial and smooth muscle cells during this period (Arras et al. 1998). The collateral growth is neither associated with perfusion deficits nor with changes in the mRNA content of hypoxia-inducible genes like LDHA. Capillary sprouting in the underperfused and partly ischemic calf muscle starts between days-5 and 7 after femoral occlusion, as demonstrated by KI67 and BrdU staining (Arras et al. 1998).

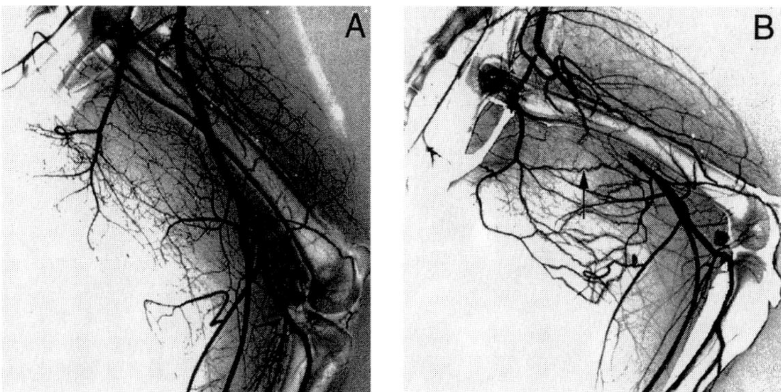

Fig. 1A,B. Postmortem angiograms of rabbit hindlimbs (**A**) without ligation of the femoral artery and (**B**) after 1 week of femoral artery occlusion. Occlusion of the femoral artery results in the development of arteries appearing in a typical corkscrew form (*arrow*)

5.3 Molecular Mechanisms

From previous studies on capillary formation it is well known that growth factors and cytokines play an important role in vessel growth. Their action is either triggered by ischemia (hypoxia) or by shear stress. To analyze the mechanisms behind arteriogenesis, we decided to characterize the function of distinct factors.

5.3.1 VEGF, an Important Angiogenic Factor, is not Directly Involved in Arteriogenesis

VEGF (reviewed by Thomas 1996), also identified as vascular permeability factor (VPF), is known to be an important angiogenic factor. It is an endothelial-specific mitogen that has been shown to be involved in both adaptive and tumor angiogenesis. The growth factor exists as four isoforms produced by alternative splicing of mRNA encoded by one gene. VEGF (or VEGF-A) is upregulated under hypoxic and ischemic conditions in vitro (Shweiki et al. 1992) and in vivo (Tudor et al. 1995), on both transcriptional and translational levels (Ikeda et al. 1995). The signal transduction proceeds via two receptor tyrosine kinases which

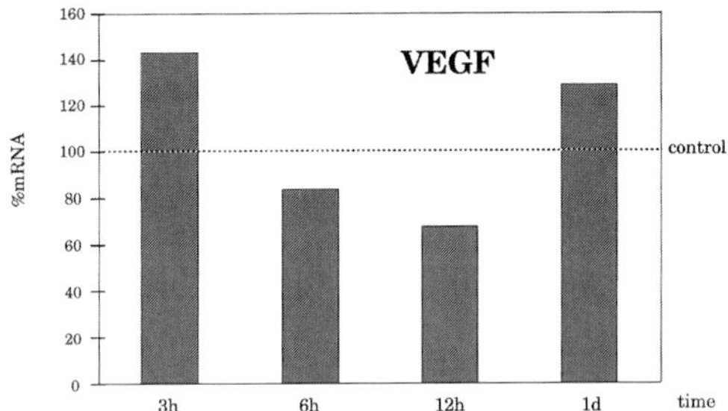

Fig. 2. Bar graphs showing the expression of VEGF mRNA in the quadriceps during the first 24 h after occlusion of the femoral artery. The VEGF mRNA was quantified by means of Northern blot analysis. Control values were defined as 100%

bind VEGF with high affinity. The VEGF receptor 1, Flt-1, is expressed on endothelial cells as well as on monocytes (Clauss et al. 1996) and has been identified as a mediator of monocyte recruitment and procoagulant activity. Flt-1 binds VEGF with about tenfold higher activity than Flk-1, the second VEGF receptor, but is only weakly tyrosine phosphorylated upon ligand binding. Flk-1, which is only expressed on endothelial cells is, in contrast, rapidly autophosphorylated on tyrosine after ligand binding, and PLCγ and MAP kinase have been shown to be phosphorylated. Binding of VEGF to Flk-1 results in signal transduction for mitogenicity, chemotaxis, and cytoskeletal reorganization (Waltenberg et al. 1996). Like VEGF Flk-1 is upregulated under hypoxic conditions on the transcriptional level in vivo (Tudor et al. 1995) and on the protein and functional level in vitro (Waltenberg et al. 1996).

Provided that angiogenesis and arteriogenesis obey one and the same mechanism, one would also expect VEGF to play an important role in collateral growth. To elucidate this point, we analyzed the expression of VEGF and its receptors using our rabbit model. After occlusion of the femoral artery, total RNA was isolated at distinct intervals from skeletal muscle of the upper leg (quadriceps, adductor) and the lower leg (gastrocenemius), and from newly developed arteries. Northern blot results revealed no significant upregulation in the expression of VEGF mRNA during the first 24 h of occlusion in the nonischemic muscles (quadriceps, adductor) where the collateral growth takes place (Fig. 2). Only in

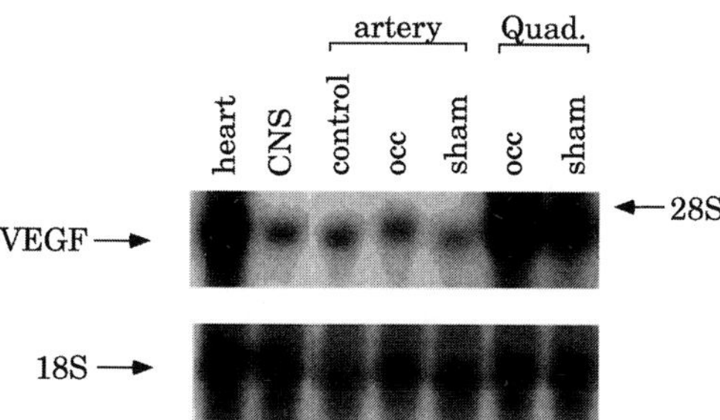

Fig. 3. Northern blot analysis of VEGF. Total RNA isolated from muscles and collateral arteries was size fractionated on a 1% agarose gel and hybridized with a cDNA probe specific for VEGF. For control purposes, we analyzed the expression of VEGF mRNA in a rabbit heart and in the CNS (central nervous system). To control RNA loading, the blot was rehybridized with an 18 S rRNA specific cDNA probe (*lower panel*). The position of the 28 S rRNA is indicated. *Quad*, quadriceps

the ischemic gastrocnemius, where sprouting of capillaries occurs, we found a significant VEGF upregulation 24 h after occlusion (Deindl et al. 1998). We analyzed the expression of VEGF mRNA in the newly developed arteries and the quadriceps 3 days after occlusion, and again found no significant change in expression (Deindl et al. 1998). Interestingly, we found that much more VEGF mRNA is expressed in the surrounding muscle than in the vessels themselves (Fig. 3), indicating that the VEGF, acting on the endothelial cells of vessels for vascular maintenance, is produced in a paracrine manner. Analyzing the mRNA expression of the two VEGF receptors, Flt-1 and Flk-1, in the same tissue/vessel samples as described above, we could not detect any significant change in the expression of either Flt-1 or Flk-1 mRNA (Deindl et al. 1998). Our data confirm that VEGF is a hypoxia-inducible factor involved in angiogenesis. At the same time, our data show that the expression of VEGF, an important angiogenic factor, is not induced in arteriogenesis, indicating that VEGF does not play a role in arteriogenesis. Although we did not analyze the expression of VEGF at the protein level, it is unlikely that VEGF acts in an autocrine or paracrine manner (supplied by monocytes) during arteriogenesis. It is known that VEGF induces the expression of its receptors at the mRNA level. An increased mRNA level for Flt-1 or Flk-1 could not be detected in our studies, contradicting an increased amount of VEGF at the protein level. In vivo data showing enhanced collateral formation after application of VEGF or induction of VEGF expression (Van Belle et al. 1998) presumably stem from the chemotactic effect of VEGF on monocytes, which – in their activated form – are supposed to play a key role in arteriogenesis (Arras et al. 1998).

5.3.2 Does the TIE System Play a Role in Arteriogenesis?

Besides the VEGF receptors, there is another family of endothelial specific transmembrane receptors comprising the TIE/TEC family (for review, see Jones 1997). Whereas the ligands for the TIE-1 receptor are unknown, two ligands are characterized for TIE-2, also called TEK: angiopoietin-1 (TIE-2 ligand 1) and angiopoietin-2 (TIE-2 ligand 2). Like VEGF, angiopoietin-1 is essential for normal vascular development in the mouse. However, it is only a weak mitogen for endothelial cells and appears to play a role in the recruitment of perivascular cells. So VEGF, with its mitogenic activity, and angiopoietin-1, exerting a chemotactic effect, act synergistically to induce sprout formation (Koblizek et al. 1998). Angiopoietin-2, on the other hand, is a naturally occurring antagonist for angiopoietin-1 and interferes with the kinase activity of TIE-2 (Hanahan 1997).

To characterize the role of the TIE/angiopoietin system in arteriogenesis, we analyzed mRNA expression of TIE-2, the TIE-2 ligand 1, and the TIE-2 ligand 2 during the first 24 h after occlusion of the femoral artery in the quadriceps and after 3 days in the quadriceps and the newly developed arteries. Northern blot analysis displayed only a very faint signal for TIE-2 in the muscle and artery samples, whereas we saw a stronger signal in the heart, which was analyzed for control purposes. For the TIE-2 ligand 1, we found significant induction in the quadriceps after 3 and 12 h of occlusion. Since we observed comparable induction in the sham operated animals, the mRNA increase of the TIE-2 ligand 1 seems not to be specific for arteriogenesis. The expression of the antagonist of the TIE-2 ligand 1, the TIE-2 ligand 2, was analyzed in the same tissue samples as that of the TIE-2 ligand 1. For this ligand, we found no change in mRNA expression in any sample

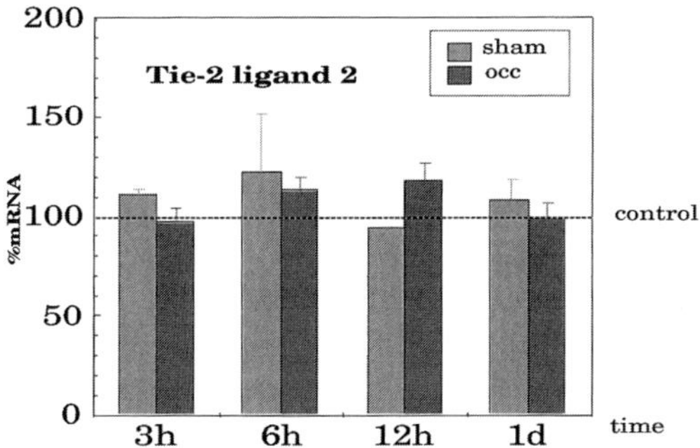

Fig. 4. Bar graphs representing the expression of the TIE-2 ligand 2 mRNA in the quadriceps during the first 24 h after occlusion of the femoral artery (*occ*) and in sham operated animals. Quantification of the mRNA levels was performed by means of Northern blot. The average of the mRNA values of non-sham operated control animals was defined as 100%. Error bars = SEM

analyzed (for an example, see Fig. 4). Although we did not analyze the protein level of the ligands and the receptor, or the degree of phosphorylation of TIE-2, it is unlikely that the TIE system plays a role in arteriogenesis. Besides our mRNA data, the facts that angiopoietin-1 (a) acts synergistically with VEGF, and (b) plays a central role in elaborating the vascular tree – not necessary for the enlargement of preexisting arterioles – make a function in this type of vessel growth unlikely.

Folkman proposed a model for the recruitment of mesenchymal cells to developing cells (Folkman and D'Amore 1996). Mesenchymal cells release angiopoietin-1, which binds to the TIE-2 receptor on endothelial cells. Activation of the receptor, in turn, leads to the production and release of a signal that recruits mesenchymal cells to the forming vessel. Upon contact, TGFβ is activated, causing mesenchymal cells to differentiate into pericytes and smooth muscle cells. We analyzed the expression of TGFβ expression in the quadriceps and in the ischemic gastrocnemius, and found increased mRNA expression in the gastrocnemius 12 and 24 h, respectively, after occlusion of the femoral artery. In the quadriceps, we found no change in expression of TGFβ during the first 24 h.

5.3.3 Increased FGFR-1 Expression is a Prerequisite for Angiogenesis and Collateral Growth

In contrast to the above mentioned endothelial cell specific receptors, the receptors of fibroblast growth factors (FGFs) are expressed on endothelial cells and smooth muscle cells. These high affinity receptors (FGFRs) are a family of structurally related, membrane-associated tyrosine kinases (Burgess and Maciag 1989). So far, four members of this family, deriving from separate genes, have been identified (Partanen et al. 1992; Fernig and Gallagher 1994). For FGFR-1 and FGFR-2, a multitude of either cell-bound or secreted isoforms have been characterized. The gene structure of these glycoproteins revealed two mechanisms responsible for the formation of diverse forms: alternative splicing, resulting in deletions or alternative exon usage, and internal polyadenylation, leading to truncated products (Givol and Yayon 1992). The expression of an isoform is tissue- and development-specific, but a single cell can express more than one isoform at once (Givol and Yayon 1992; Jin et al. 1994). Ligand-induced dimerization of the FGFRs is a key event in transmembrane signaling. It results in autophosphorylation and the induction of diverse biological responses (Schlessinger and Ullrich 1992; Schlessinger et al. 1995). FGFR-1 mRNA is the predominant form of the four known FGFRs expressed by proliferating smooth muscle cells (Xin et al. 1994). This strongly suggests that this is the type of FGFR that mediates signal transduction in proliferating smooth muscle cells.

To analyze the role of FGFR-1 in arteriogenesis compared to angiogenesis, we again analyzed mRNA expression of the receptor in the growing arteries, in the nonischemic quadriceps and adductor, and the ischemic gastrocnemius. The results displayed a very rapid increase of this mRNA (3 h after occlusion) in all muscle samples analyzed. However, this increase was much more pronounced in muscle regions where collateral growth takes place (Fig. 5). Peak levels at 6 h of occlusion of the femoral artery were followed by a continuous decrease towards control value 3 days after occlusion. Although the increase of the FGFR-1 mRNA was not as prominent in the ischemic gastrocnemius, the decline towards control values did not proceed as drastically as in the nonischemic upper leg. Our results indicate that both angiogenesis and arteriogenesis are dependent on increased expression of FGFR-1. This

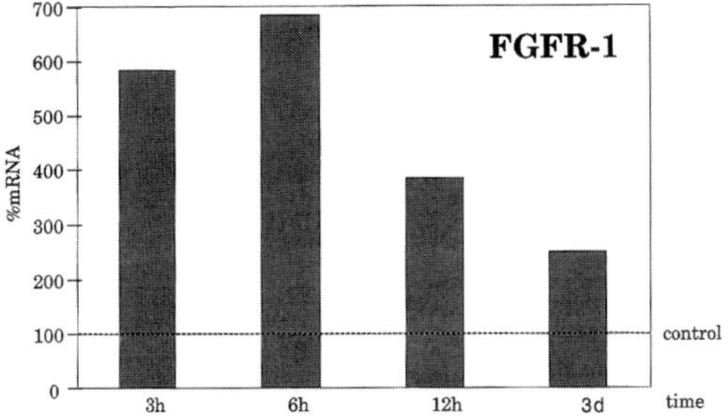

Fig. 5. Bar graphs showing expression of the FGFR-1 mRNA in the quadriceps during the first 24 h after occlusion of the femoral artery. The quantification of the FGFR-1 mRNA was performed by means of Northern blot analysis. Control values were defined as 100%

implies that the effect of therapeutically applied FGFs might be further enhanced by stimulating expression of FGFR-1 (Deindl et al. 1997).

5.3.3.1 Syndecan-4 and uPA are Possibly Involved in FGFR-1 Activation

Activation of cells by FGFs involves not only high-affinity receptor kinases, but also low-affinity receptors consisting of a small core protein, the so-called proteoglycans, and an attached glycosaminoglycan (GAG) (Jackson et al. 1991). The most important GAGs for FGFs are heparin and heparan sulfate. Heparin binds simultaneously to a number of FGFs, resulting in their oligomerization. Upon release of the complex by proteases, multivalent binding of the multimeric FGF complex to the high-affinity receptor stimulates FGFR dimerization and activation (Fig. 6) (Spivak-Kroizman et al. 1994; Schlessinger et al. 1995). Facilitation of the FGF-FGFR interaction by heparan sulfate was evidenced by high-affinity binding of FGF-2 to heparan sulfate proteoglycan (Moscatelli 1987) and by the observation that heparan-sulfate-proteoglycan-deficient cells fail to show FGF-R dimerization or tyrosine kinase activation (Spivak-Kroizman et al. 1994). Cell surface proteoglycans are ubiquitous components of the plasma membranes of mammalian cells.

Our interest focused on the syndecans, a group of proteoglycans that bind actin inside the cell and growth factors plus the extracellular matrix

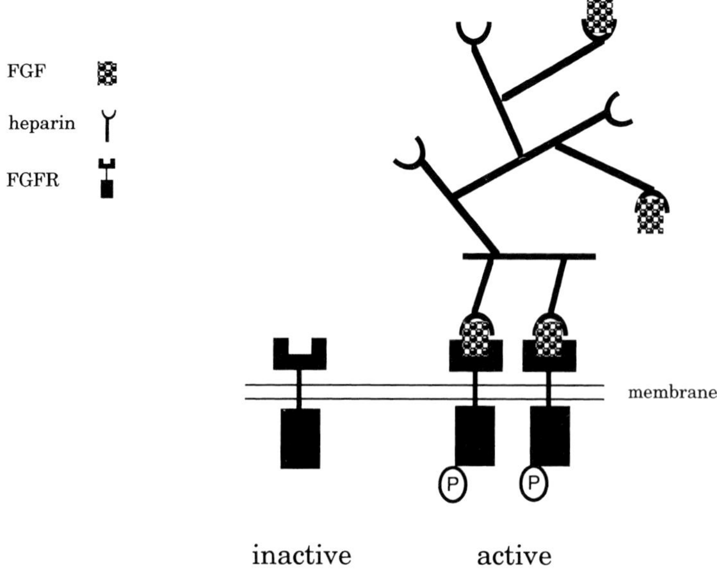

Fig. 6. A scheme for activation of a FGFR by interaction with a multimeric FGF-heparin sulfate proteoglycan complex. A cell-surface proteoglycan molecule binds simultaneously to several FGF molecules, which in turn bind to the signaling FGFR. Multivalent binding of the FGF complex stimulates FGFR dimerization and activation. *P*, phosphorylated tyrosine kinase residue

outside the cell (Saunders and Bernfield 1988; Elenius et al. 1992; Salmivirta et al. 1992). Currently, four syndecans – each bearing three covalently attached heparan sulfates – have been characterized (Woods and Couchman 1998). There is a variability in the spatial and temporal expression of syndecans. In adult tissue, syndecan-1, -2, and -3 are the major syndecans in epithelial cells, fibroblasts, and neuronal cells, respectively. Syndecan-4, by contrast, is usually present in lower amounts than the major syndecan species but more widespread in distribution. Syndecan-4 co-localizes with integrins at focal adhesions but can also bind to and activate PKC. (Waltenberg et al. 1996) Analyzing the expression of syndecans in our animal model, we found a pronounced mRNA increase of syndecan-4 in the upper leg 3 h after occlusion of the femoral artery (Fig. 7). Although there was minor induction in sham

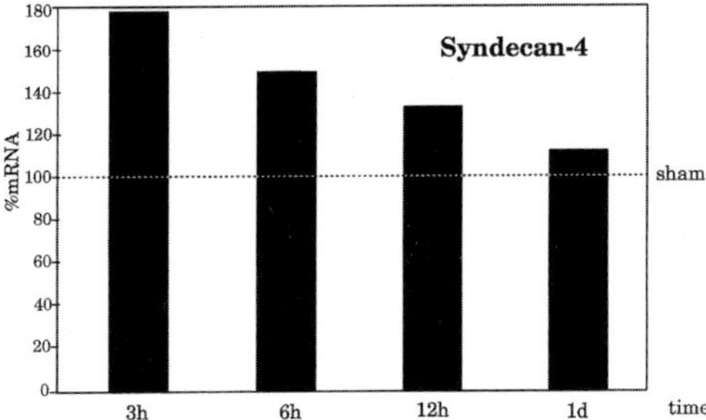

Fig. 7. Bar graphs showing the expression of the syndecan-4 mRNA in the quadriceps during the first 24 h after occlusion of the femoral artery. Quantification of the mRNA levels was performed by means of Northern blot. The average of the mRNA values of sham operated animals was defined as 100%

operated animals, our results indicate that this proteoglycan is involved in collateral growth.

Controlled extracellular proteolysis is catalyzed in part by the secretion of plasminogen activators. The serine proteases convert plasminogen into the active protease plasmin. Two types of plasminogen activators have been identified: the tissue-type plasminogen activator (tPA) (Astrup and Permin 1947) and the urokinase-type plasminogen activator (uPA) (Williams 1951). Plasminogen activators are synthesized by a number of cells, and actively regulated by hormones and many other agents (Ny et al. 1988). Enzyme production has been correlated with several processes involving cell migration and tissue remodeling (Vassalli and Reich 1977; Gross et al. 1982; Ossowski and Reich 1983). Plasminogen activator induction can result from either urokinase (Nagamine et al. 1983; Belin et al. 1984) or tissue plasminogen activator mRNA content (Opdenakker et al. 1983). In addition, plasminogen activator activity can be modulated at post-translational levels, including the secretion of the enzyme (Belin et al. 1984) and the concomitant production of plasminogen activator specific protease inhibitors (Vassalli et al. 1984). In our model we analyzed the expression of uPA, which has already been shown to be upregulated in pig myocardium during coronary artery occlusion (Knoepfler et al. 1995). We analyzed the expression of uPA mRNA during the first 24 h after occlusion of the femoral artery in the quadriceps. Whereas we found strong induction in

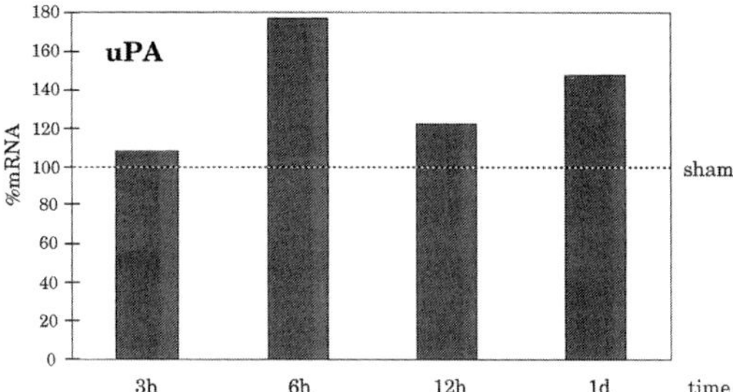

Fig. 8. Bar graphs showing the expression of the uPA mRNA in the quadriceps during the first 24 h after femoral occlusion. Quantification of the mRNA levels was performed by means of Northern blot. The average of the mRNA values of sham operated animals was defined as 100%

the experimental tissue as well as in the tissue from sham operated animals 3 h after occlusion, we found significant induction 6 h after occlusion, but only in the experimental tissue, indicating that this was a specific response to femoral ligation (Fig. 8). Although syndecan-4, as well as uPA, might be involved in low-affinity, receptor-mediated activation of the FGFR-1, we can not exclude the possibility that upregulation of the corresponding mRNAs is due to another, still uncharacterized mechanism involved in arteriogenesis.

5.3.3.2 Unchanged Expression of bFGF in the Growing Arteries

The ligands of FGFRs comprise a family consisting of at least 15 heparin-binding polypeptide growth factors. They mediate a broad range of biological activities (hematopoiesis, development, wound repair, angiogenesis) in a variety of cell types of mesenchymal and neuroectodermal origin (Baird and Klagsbrunn 1991; Givol and Yayon 1992; Fernig and Gallagher 1994). aFGF and bFGF, preferentially bound by the FGFR-1, are potent mitogens and play an important role in cell proliferation and differentiation (Burgess and Maciag 1989; Basilico and Moscatelli 1992; Johnson and Wiliams 1993; Jin et al. 1994; Wang et al. 1994). They lack hydrophobic signal peptides and are therefore concentrated within their cell of origin (Abraham et al. 1986). However, both growth factors are also found in the extracellular matrix and basement membranes of a variety of embryonic and adult tissues. Up to now, their manner of secretion is unknown, but it is obvious that it is different from classical secretion (McNeil et al. 1989; Muthukrishan et al. 1991; Mignatti et al. 1992).

For each ligand various isoforms are known, which either result from alternative splicing (aFGF) (Myers et al. 1993) or initiation of translation either at an internal AUG codon or at CUG codons 5' of the AUG codon (Florkiewicz and Sommer 1989; Prats et al. 1989). While looking for the mRNA expression of aFGF and bFGF, we did not find any significant change, either in the quadriceps or in growing arteries (Deindl et al. 1997). Because macrophages play a key role in angiogenesis, we focused on the idea that growth factors and other monokines might be supplied to the growing arteries by macrophages.

5.3.4 The Importance of Monocytes and Macrophages

The importance of macrophages derives from their ubiquitous presence in tissue, their potential to become activated in response to appropriate stimuli, and their repertoire of secretory products. Analyzing the infiltration of monocytes in our animal model, we found adhesion of these mononuclear cells to the endothelium of the growing arteries as early as 12 h after occlusion (D. Scholz, personal communication). Progressive and massive accumulation in the adventita of an arteriole was seen up to day-3 after occlusion (Arras et al. 1998). Monocyte accumulation was also observed in the gastrocnemius where capillary sprouting occurs. However, tissue macrophages were not seen to accumulate until day-7 after occlusion, correlating with the late appearance of capillary proliferation in the lower limb. Double staining of excised collaterals for macrophages and bFGF revealed that this growth factor is almost exclusively found in monocytes. In contrast to the upper leg, positive staining for bFGF in the ischemic lower leg was not confined to macrophages but was also seen in many other cells (Arras et al. 1998). Our results indicate that monocytes play an important role not only in angiogenesis but also in arteriogenesis – at least via supplying growth factors.

Adhesion of monocytes on the endothelial cell layer of a vessel requires the expression of cell adhesion molecules. Analyzing the expression of the intercellular cell adhesion molecule (ICAM) and vascular cell adhesion molecule (VCAM), we found an increased mRNA

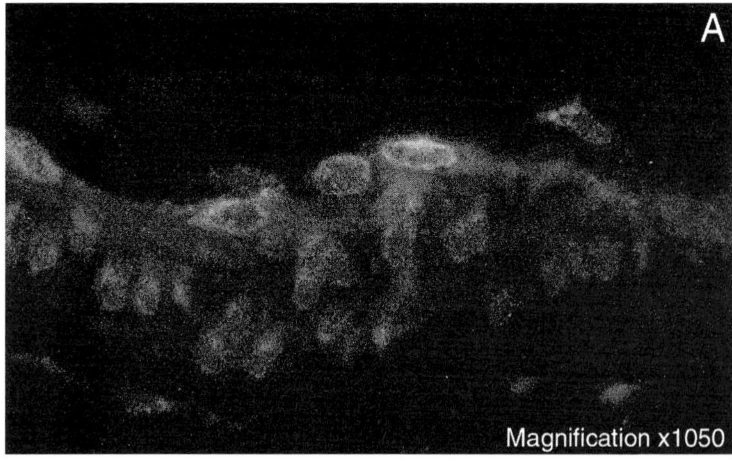

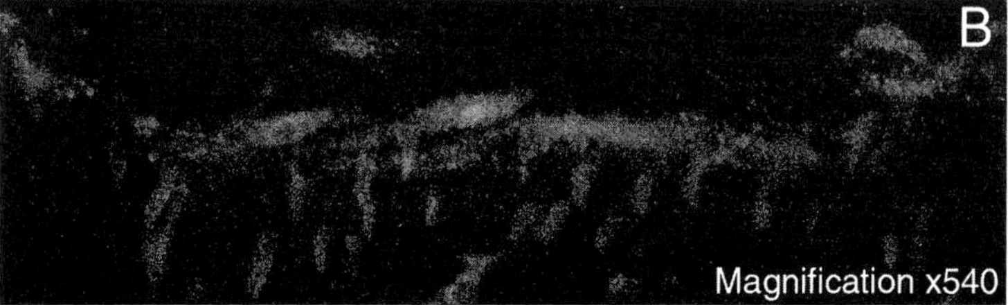

Fig. 9A,B. Immunohistochemical staining for ICAM-1 and VCAM-1 in the upper leg. The picture shows a positive reaction for ICAM-1 (**A**) and VCAM-1 (**B**) in endothelial cells of a growing collateral artery 2 days after occlusion of the femoral artery (Courtesy of D. Scholz)

level for both transcripts 12 h after occlusion of the artery. Immunohistochemical data confirmed these results (Fig. 9). A first positive reaction to ICAM and VCAM staining was recognized 12 h after occlusion, the earliest time when infiltrated monocytes could be proven (D. Scholz, personal communication). This suggests that, in our model, ICAM and VCAM are involved in the adhesion of monocytes.

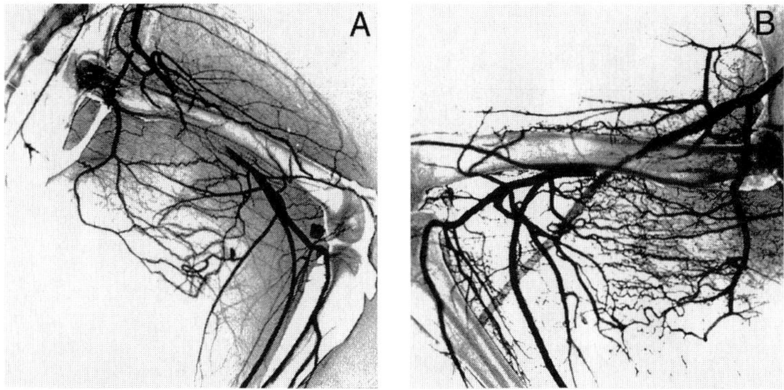

Fig. 10A,B. Postmortem angiograms of rabbit hindlimbs after 7 days of femoral artery occlusion without MCP-1 treatment (**A**) and after 1 week of local MCP-1 infusion (**B**). The density of collateral vessels with typical corkscrew appearance is markedly increased in hindlimbs treated with MCP-1

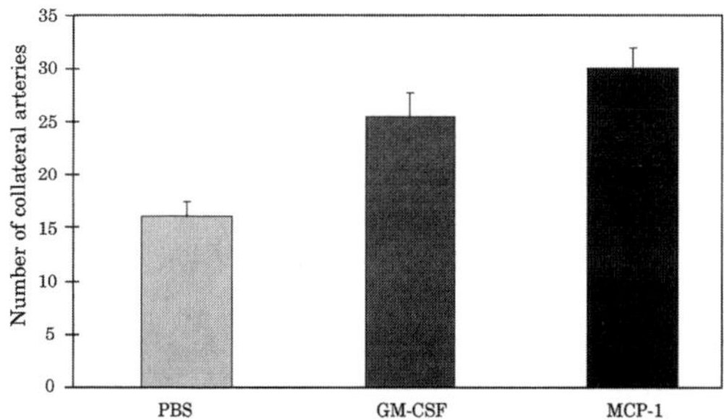

Fig. 11. Bar graphs representing the number of visible collateral arteries in a rabbit hindlimb with occluded femoral artery after 1 week of local infusion of PBS, GM-CSF, or MCP-1. Error bars = SEM. (Courtesy of I. Höfer)

5.3.5 MCP-1 and GM-CSF Promote Collateral Growth

On the basis of this finding, we were interested in knowing whether collateral artery growth can be promoted by inducing monocyte chemotaxis – via the application of MCP-1 (monocyte chemoattractant protein-1) – or by activating and prolonging the survival of the involved macrophages via application of the granulocyte-macrophage colony-stimulating factor (GM-CSF) . In vivo, the infusion of MCP-1 (Fig. 10) and of GM-CSF (Fig. 11) resulted in increased collateral conductance and enhanced arteriogenesis (Ito et al. 1997; Buschmann et al. 1998). The results emphasize the importance of macrophages in arteriogenesis and make MCP-1 and GM-CSF candidates for therapeutic purposes.

5.4 Conclusions

Understanding the molecular mechanisms of collateral formation should provide the tools for inducing and enhancing collateral growth in human patients. Vascular growth in the adult organism proceeds either via capillary sprouting or by in situ enlargement of preexisting arteriolar connections into collateral arteries. However, it remained unclear whether collateral growth and capillary sprouting, also called angiogenesis, depend on one and the same or two distinct molecular mechanisms. Analyzing the molecular dynamics behind arteriogenesis and angiogenesis, we received strong indications that both types of vessel growth do not follow the same patterns. Being an important angiogenic factor, VEGF does not seem to be directly involved in arteriogenesis. bFGF and FGFR-1 are supposed to play a role in both mechanisms, whereby bFGF is supplied during angiogenesis in an autocrine and paracrine way, and with arteriogenesis only in a paracrine manner.

Activated monocytes play a key role in arteriogenesis, presumably in their ability to release growth factors and cytokines responsible for vessel growth. The ability to attract and activate monocytes, as shown by the application of MCP-1 and GM-CSF, might be in important step towards enhancing artery growth.

Acknowledgement. We thank *Circulation Research* for giving us permission to reproduce a picture (Ito et al. 1997).

References

Abraham JA, Mergia A, Whang JL, Tumola A, Gospodarowicz D, Fiddes JC (1986) Nucleotide sequence of a bovine clone encoding the angiogenic protein, basic fibroblast growth factor. Science 233:545–548

Arras M, Ito WD, Scholz D, Winkler B, Schaper J, Schaper W (1998) Monocyte activation in angiogenesis and collateral growth in the rabbit hindlimb. J Clin Invest 101(1):40–50

Astrup T, Permin PM (1947) Fibrinolysis of the animal organism. Nature 159:681–682

Baird A, Klagsbrunn M (1991) The fibroblast growth factor family. Cancer Cells 3(6):239–243

Basilico C, Moscatelli D (1992) The FGF family of growth factors and oncogenes. Adv Cancer Res 59:115–165

Belin D, Godeau F, Vassilli JD (1984) Tumor promoter PMA stimulates the synthesis and secretion of mouse pro-urokinase in MSV-transformed 3T3 cells: this is mediated by an increase in urokinase mRNA content. EMBO J 3(8):1901–1906

Burgess WH, Maciag T (1989) The heparin-binding (fibroblast) growth factor family of proteins. Annu Rev Biochem 58:575–606

Buschmann I, Ito W, Höfer I, Weiß G, Kostin S, Schaper J, Schaper W (1998) GM-CSF promotes collateral artery growth via prolongation of macrophage survival. J Mol Cell Cardiol 30:A126 (abstract)

Clauss M, Weich H, Breier G, Knies U, Roeckl W, Waltenberg J, Risau W (1996) The vascular endothelial growth factor receptor Flt-1 mediates biological activities. J Biol Chem 271:17629–17634

Deindl E, Ito W, Zimmermann R, Schaper W (1997) Increased FGFR1 expression is a prerequisite for angiogenesis and collateral growth. J Mol Med 75(5):13 (abstract)

Deindl E, Ito W, Zimmermann RJ, Schaper W (1998) VEGF, in important angiogenic factor, is not involved in arteriogenesis. J Mol Med 76(6):B24 (abstract)

Elenius K, Maatta A, Salmivirta M, Jalkanen M (1992) Growth factors induce 3T3 cells to express bFGF-binding syndecan. J Biol Chem 267(9):6435–6441

Fernig DG, Gallagher JT (1994) Fibroblast growth factors and their receptors: an information network controlling tissue growth, morphogenesis and repair. Prog Growth Factor Res 5:353–377

Florkiewicz RZ, Sommer D (1989) Human basic fibroblast growth factor gene encodes four polypeptides: three initiate translation from non-AUG codons. Proc Natl Acad Sci USA 86:3978–3981

Folkman J (1995) Tumor angiogenesis. Saunders, Philadelphia

Folkman J, D'Amore PA (1996) Blood vessel formation: what is its molecular basis. Cell 87:1153–1155

Givol D, Yayon A (1992) Complexity of FGF receptors: genetic basis for structural diversity and functional specificity. FASEB 6:3362–3369

Görge G, Schmidt T, Ito BR, Pantely G, Schaper W (1988) Microvascular and collateral adaptation in swine hearts following progressive coronary artery stenosis. Basic Res Cardiol 84:524–535

Gross JL, Moscatelli D, Jaffe EA, Rifkin DB (1982) Plasminogen activator and collagenase production by cultured capillary endothelial cells. J Cell Biol 95:974–981

Hanahan D (1997) Signaling vascular morphogenesis and maintenance. Science 277:48–50

Ikeda E, Achen MG, Breier G, Risau W (1995) Hypoxia-induced transcriptional activation and increased mRNA stability of vascular endothelial growth factor in C6 glioma cells. J Biol Chem 270:19761–19766

Isner JM, Piezcek A, Schainfeld R, Blair R, Haley L, Asahara T, Rosenfield K, Razvi S, Walsh K, Symes JF (1996) Clinical evidence of angiogenesis after arterial gene transfer of phVEGF165 in patient with ischaemic limb. Lancet 348:370–374

Ito WD, Arras M, Winkler B, Scholz D, Schaper J, Schaper W (1997) Monocyte chemotactic protein-1 increases collateral and peripheral conductance after femoral artery occlusion. Circ Res 80:829–837

Jackson RL, Busch SJ, Cardin AD (1991) Glycosaminoglycans molecular properties protein interactions and role in physiological processes. Physiol Rev 71:481–540

Jin Y, Pasumarthi BS, Bock ME, Lytras A, Kardami E, Cattini PA (1994) Cloning and expression of fibroblast growth factor receptor-1 isoforms in the mouse heart: evidence for isoform switching during heart development. J Mol Cell Cardiol 26:1449–1459

Johnson DE, Williams LT (1993) Structural and functional diversity in the FGF receptor multigene family growth factors and oncogenes. Adv Cancer Res 60:1–60

Jones PF (1997) Tied up (or down?) with angiopoietins. Angiogenesis 1(1):38–44

Knoepfler PS, Bloor CM, Carroll SM (1995) Urokinase plasminogen activator activity is increased in the myocardium during coronary artery occlusion. J Mol Cell Cardiol 27:1317–1324

Koblizek TI, Weis C, Yancpoulos GD, Deutsch U, Risau W (1998) Angiopoietin induces sprouting angiogenesis in-vitro. Curr Biol 8(N9):529–532

McNeil PL, Muthukrishnan WE, D'Amore PA (1989) Growth factors are released by mechanically wounded endothelial cells. J Cell Biol 109:811–821

Mignatti P, Morimoto T, Rifkin DB (1992) Basic fibroblast growth factor, a protein devoid of of secretory signal sequence, is released by cells via a pathway independent of the endoplasmic reticulum-Golgi complex. J Cell Physiol 151:81–93

Moscatelli D (1987) High and low affinity binding sites for basic fibroblast growth factor on cultured cells absence of a role for low affinity binding in the stimulation of plasminogen activator production by bovine capillary endothelial cells. J Cell Physiol 131(1):123–130

Muthukrishan L, Warder E, McNeil PL (1991) Basic fibroblast growth factor is efficiently released from cytosolic storage sites through plasma membrane disruptions of endothelial cells. J Cell Physiol 148:1–16

Myers RL, Payson RA, Chotani MA, Deaven LL, Chiu IM (1993) Gene structure and differential expression of acidic fibroblast growth factor mRNA: identification and distribution of four different transcripts. Oncogene 8(2):341–349

Nagamine Y, Sudol M, Reich E (1983) Hormonal regulation of plasminogen activator mRNA in porcine kidney cells. Cell 32(4):1184–1190

Ny T, Ohlsson M, Strandberg L (1988) The gene for t-PA in tissue-type plasminogen activator (t-PA). In: Kluft C (ed) Physiological and clinical aspects. CRC Press, Boca Raton

Opdenakker G, Ashino-Fuse H, Van Damme J, Billiau A, De Somer P (1983) Effects of 12-O-tetradecanoylphorbol 13-acetate on the production of mRNAs for human tissue-type plasminogen activator. Eur J Biochem 131:481–487

Ossowski L, Reich E (1983) Antibodies to plasminogen activator inhibit human tumor metastasis. Cell 35:611–619

Partanen J, Vainikka S, Korhonen J, Armstrong E, Alitalo K (1992) Diverse receptors for fibroblast growth factors. Prog Growth Factors Res 4(1):69–83

Plate KH, Breier G, Weich HA, Risau W (1992) Vascular endothelial growth factor is a potential tumor angiogenesis factor in human gliomas in vivo. Nature 359:845–848

Prats H, Kaghad M, Prats AC, Klagsbrun M, Lelias JM, Liauzun P, Chalon P, Tauber JP, Amalric F, Smith JA, Caput D (1989) High molecular mass forms of basic fibroblast growth factor are initiated by alternative CUG codons. Proc Natl Acad Sci USA 86:1836–1840

Salmivirta M, Heino J, Jalkanen M (1992) Basic fibroblast growth factor syndecan complex at cell surface or immobilized to matrix promotes cell growth. J Biol Chem 267(25):17606–17610

Saunders S, Bernfield M (1988) Cell surface proteoglycan binds mouse mammary epithelial cells to fibronectin and behaves as a receptor for intestinal matrix. J Cell Biol 106(2):423–430

Schaper W, Schaper J (1993) Collateral circulation – heart, brain, kidney, limbs. Kluwer Academic, Boston

Schlessinger J, Ullrich A (1992) Growth factor signaling by receptor tyrosine kinases. Neuron 9:383–391

Schlessinger J, Lax I, Lemmon M (1995) Regulation of growth factor activation by proteoglycans: what is the role of the low affinity receptors? Cell 83:357–360

Shweiki D, Itin A, Soffer D, Keshet E (1992) Vascular endothelial growth factor induced by hypoxia may mediate hypoxia-initiated angiogenesis. Nature 359:843–845

Spivak-Kroizman T, Lemmon MA, Dikic I, Ladbury JE, Pinchasi D, Huang J, Jaye M, Crumley G, Schlessinger J, Lax I (1994) Heparin-induced oligomerization of FGF molecules is responsible for FGF receptor dimerization, activation, and cell proliferation. Cell 79:1015–1024

Thomas KA (1996) Vascular endothelial growth factor, a potent and selective angiogenic agent. J Biol Chem 271:603–606

Tudor RM, Flook BE, Voelkel NF (1995) Increased gene expression of VEGF and the VEGF receptors KDR/Flk and Flt in lungs exposed to acute or to chronic ischemia. J Clin Invest 95:1789–1807

Van Belle E, Witzenbichler B, Chen D, Silver M, Ling C, Isner JM (1998) Potentiated angiogenic effect of scatter factor/hepatocyte growth factor via induction of vascular endothelial growth factor. Circulation 97:381–390

Vassalli JD, Reich E (1977) Macrophage plasminogen activator: induction of products of activated lymphoid cells. J Exp Med 145:429–437

Vassalli JD, Dayer JM, Wohlwend A, Belin D (1984) Concomitant secretion of prourokinase and of a plasminogen activator-specific inhibitor by cultured human monocytes-macrophages. J Exp Med 159:1653–1668

Waltenberg J, Mayr U, Pentz S, Hombach V (1996) Functional upregulation of vascular endothelial growth factor receptor KDR by hypoxia. Circulation 94(7):1647–1654

Wang J-K, Gao G, Goldfarb M (1994) Fibroblast growth factor receptors have different signaling and mitogenic potentials. Mol Cell Biol 14(1):181–188

Williams JRB (1951) The fibrinolytic activity of urine. Br J Exp Pathol 32:530–537

Woods A, Couchman R (1998) Syndecans: synergistic acitvators of cell adhesion. Trends Cell Biol 8:189–192

Xin X, Johnson AD, Scott-Burden T, Engler D, Casscells W (1994) The predominant form of fibroblast growth factor receptor expressed by proliferating human arterial smooth muscle cells in culture is type I. Biochem Biophys Res Commun 204(2):557–564

6 Hemodynamic Forces, Exercise, and Angiogenesis

O. Hudlická, M. D. Brown

6.1 Introduction

It is generally acknowledged that training results in capillary growth in skeletal muscle, with the extent of growth varying according to length and type of training. There is also growth of arterioles and expansion of the whole vascular bed, as indicated by increased maximal conductance. Surprisingly, in the heart, training results in capillary growth almost predominantly in young animals, while growth of arterioles and enlargement of large vessels occurs in adults, even when not accompanied by capillary growth (see Hudlická et al. 1992). There is no doubt that the changes in capillary supply are due at least in part to growth of endothelial cells, which was demonstrated by [^{3}H]thymidine incorporation in capillary nuclei in the hearts of animals trained by swimming (Mandache et al. 1973). Although there is no parallel evidence in skeletal muscles, increased capillarization demonstrated either by histochemical techniques which depict specifically capillary endothelium, or by electron microscopy, thus revealing all anatomically present vessels, are the result of growth of new vessels.

In spite of many studies on the effects of physical exercise on vascular bed growth in the heart and skeletal muscles, very little is known about the mechanisms which initiate it. A single bout of exercise was shown to increase mRNA levels for VEGF (but not bFGF) and, to a smaller extent, TGFb1 in skeletal muscle (Breen et al. 1996). Richardson et al. (1998) described a much smaller increase in muscles of trained individuals, whose capillary supply was 18% higher than in control subjects and suggested that VEGF may be involved in the initiation of capillary growth, while the signal is attenuated once capillary supply has been increased. To our knowledge, there are no corresponding data with respect to the heart.

Although growth factors are very important as stimuli of angiogenesis under pathological circumstances, mechanical factors may play a dominant role in angiogenesis elicited by physiological means such as exercise training, increased muscle activity by electrical stimulation, or long-term increase in blood flow resulting from exposure to cold or high altitude hypoxia (Hudlická et al. 1992; Hudlická and Brown 1993). We will try to establish to what extent changes in blood flow are related to angiogenesis in skeletal and cardiac muscle under different physiological circumstances and which components, such as shear stress or circumferential wall stress, may be involved. We will also show to what extent any of these physiological procedures could help improve capillary growth in ischemic muscles and the heart.

6.2 Effect of Training on Capillary Growth in Skeletal Muscle – Role of Blood Flow

Capillary growth from endurance training has been described in both men and women (see Saltin and Gollnick 1983; Hudlická et al. 1992) and is related to the intensity of activity. This was clearly demonstrated in cross-country skiers, where EMG monitoring showed greater activity and greater increases in capillary supply in the triceps brachii than in the vastus lateralis (Schantz et al. 1983). Although Schantz could not measure blood flow in this particular group, it is known to increase in relation to the intensity of dynamic exercise.

Is there any evidence that capillary growth is related to increased blood flow? Increases in capillary supply, expressed either as capillary density (CD), number of capillaries per mm^2, or capillary:fiber ratio (C:F) first occurs in the vicinity of slow and fast oxidative fibers which are already surrounded by more capillaries than fast glycolytic fibers (Gray and Renkin 1978). This has been shown in both animals (Mai et al. 1970) and humans (Ingjer 1979). Laughlin and Armstrong (1982) demonstrated preferential increases in blood flow in slow and fast oxidative muscles or their parts during exercise, while the flow in fast glycolytic muscles, which operate mainly on anaerobic metabolism, increased only during exhaustive exercise. Gute et al. (1994) showed increased capillary supply in glycolytic muscles in rats trained by sprinting, which in turn resulted in increased flow capacity (Sexton et al. 1988), while mild endurance training increased capillary:fiber ratios in muscles composed predominantly of oxidative fibers. High intensity training increased capillary supply in all muscles (Gute et al. 1996) with a relatively modest increase in flow capacity (Sexton and Laughlin 1994). In sprint-trained animals, resting blood flow before and after training was higher in the muscle group with increased capillary:fiber ratio (Laughlin et al. 1988); low intensity endurance training increased resting flow in mixed muscle and less so in the red part of the muscle in proportion to increase in the capillary:fiber ratio. So there is some correlation between changes in blood flow and capillary supply but blood flow is probably not the only relevant cause of capillary growth resulting from training.

The other important factor is change in the muscle oxidative capacity. Andersen and Henriksson (1977) demonstrated that increases in cytochrome oxidase preceded increases in capillary density in athletes who trained for 8 weeks. The latter increases were modest and smaller than those in oxidative capacity. Although capillary growth can be induced in almost any muscle with the appropriate training regime, it occurs after a relatively long period of time. So far, apart from the above-mentioned work on VEGF, there have been very few attempts to elucidate the sequence of vascular changes and factors that initiate them.

6.3 Role of Hemodynamic Factors in Capillary Growth in Skeletal Muscles Induced by Chronic Electrical Stimulation

In contrast to training, long-term increases in activity by electrical stimulation resulted in a very rapid increase in capillary supply (Brown et al. 1976; Hudlická and Tyler 1984) which was preceded by endothelial cell proliferation as shown by an increase in the labeling index for bromodeoxyuridine (BrdU) in capillary-linked nuclei (Hudlická et al. 1998a). Unlike exercise, electrical stimulation eliciting near maximal force of contraction activates all muscle fibers at the same time, which could cause the fast glycolytic fibers to become hypoxic, since their capillary supply may be inadequate for the continuous activity to which they are exposed.

If hypoxia is a stimulus for capillary growth, then any increase in capillarization should first occur in the vicinity of the affected fibers. Capillary density was indeed increased in the vicinity of fast glycolytic fibers, but no others, after only 2 days of stimulation (Hudlická et al. 1982). However, direct measurements of oxygen tension in stimulated muscles did not reveal lower values (Hudlická et al. 1984). Furthermore, hypoxia usually results in an increase in the activity of oxidative enzymes (Valdivia and Watson 1960) and higher volume density of mitochondria (Hoppeler and Desplanches 1992). However, preferential stimulation of glycolytic fibers using low intensity current increased capillary:fiber ratios in the glycolytic part of the tibialis anterior, without changes in cytochrome oxidase activity (Egginton and Hudlická 1989). Finally, when the blood supply of stimulated muscles was limited by ligation of the common iliac artery, the volume density of mitochondria increased to a similar degree as in stimulated muscles with normal blood supply, but without increases in the capillary:fiber ratio (Hudlická

1991). All this evidence indicates that hypoxia does not initiate capillary growth in chronically stimulated muscles, possibly not even in trained ones, and that an increase in blood flow is essential for this process.

Could the preferential increase in capillary growth near glycolytic fibers be explained by changes in blood flow? Although blood flow in resting muscles composed predominantly of fast glycolytic fibers is low, it can increase more during muscle contractions (Hudlická 1975) and high speed running (Armstrong and Laughlin 1983) than the flow in fast or slow oxidative muscles.

The differential change in blood flow was also shown on the capillary level. With the onset of contractions, the velocity of red blood cells (Vrbc) increased more rapidly and to a greater extent in capillaries supplying the superficial layer of the rat tibialis anterior, composed mainly of glycolytic fibers, than in those supplying purely oxidative soleus (Dawson et al. 1987). The role of blood flow as a stimulus for capillary growth was further demonstrated by the fact that long-term administration of various vasodilators resulted in increased capillary supply (Hudlická 1991; Hudlická et al. 1992).

How can increased blood flow or increased Vrbc induce capillary growth? Higher Vrbc would result in higher shear stress, provided the capillary diameters do not appreciably change, since shear stress (τ) is directly proportional to Vrbc and indirectly proportional to capillary radius (*r*) [$\tau=\eta\times(4\text{Vrbc}/r)$]. It is also directly proportional to viscosity (η). This is, in turn, related to hematocrit, which is higher in contracting than in resting muscles (Duling and Desjardins 1987). Direct measurements of diameter and Vrbc in capillaries supplying the glycolytic part of the tibialis anterior at rest and during contraction (Dawson 1987) showed that calculated shear stress increased by 75% (Hudlická et al. 1998b) and was higher even at rest in muscles that had been stimulated for 7 days (Dawson and Hudlická 1993), although hematocrit was considered to be similar in resting and contracting muscles (Table 1).

Shear stress is known to stimulate endothelial proliferation in tissue cultures (Ando et al. 1987). It has also been established that it causes release of prostaglandins and nitric oxide from endothelium in vivo (Koller and Kaley 1996). Although the results on the role of NO as a stimulus for endothelial cell growth are controversial (Pilipi-Synetos et al. 1995; Ziche et al. 1994), there is no doubt that prostaglandins induce capillary growth (Ben Ezra 1978; Form and Auerbach 1983). Long-term

Table 1. Capillary shear stress in contracting and stimulated muscles

	Capillary diameter	Vrbc (μm/s)	Calculated shear stress dyne/cm^2
Control at rest	3.3±0.1	259±60	12.50±2.81
Control at 1 Hz	3.6±0.1	439±77*	19.58±3.67
S7	3.4±0.1	420±60*	18.84±2.57

Capillary diameters, velocity of red blood cells (Vrbc) and calculated shear stress [$\tau=\eta\times(4\text{Vrbc}/r)$] (mean±SEM) in capillaries on the surface of tibialis anterior muscle at rest and during contractions at 1 Hz in control muscles, and at rest (at least 16 h after the termination of stimulation) in muscles that were stimulated for 7 days, 8 h/day at 10 Hz (S7). Data from 25–30 vessels in each group. (From Dawson 1987; Dawson and Hudlická 1993)
*$p<0.05$ versus control

administration of the cyclooxygenase inhibitor indomethacin (Pearce and Hudlická 1995) and the nitric oxide synthase inhibitor L-NNA (Hudlická et al. 1996) indeed suppressed increases in the labeling index for BrdU and the C:F ratio in stimulated muscles.

Increased blood flow could also lead to changes in capillary pressure and, thus increased capillary wall tension, which in turn could result in disturbance of the basement membrane and, therefore, release of growth factors. Although the capillary diameters are only marginally wider in contracting (Dawson 1987) or chronically stimulated muscles (Dawson and Hudlická 1989), arterioles are significantly wider after only 2 days of stimulation (Table 2). This could result in increased capillary pressure and thus wall tension in stimulated muscles, even at rest. Moreover, capillary pressure is known to be considerably higher during muscle contractions (Mellander and Bjornberg 1992), which also contributes to the increase in wall tension (Dawson and Hudlická 1993; Hudlická et al. 1998a). Although arteriolar diameters return to control values in muscles that had been stimulated for 7 days, higher capillary pressure in the early stages of stimulation and in muscles that contract for 8 h a day should be considered as another hemodynamic factor possibly involved in the initiation of capillary growth.

There are signs of basement membrane disturbance in muscles that had been stimulated for 4 but not for 2 days, as demonstrated by electron microscopy (Hansen-Smith et al. 1996). However, the basic fibroblast

Table 2. Diameters of arterioles and venules (in μm) in stimulated muscles

	Control	Stimulated for 2 days	Stimulated for 7 days
A3	8.0±0.2	9.2±0.5*	7.4±0.2
A4	5.6±0.1	6.6±0.2*	5.7±0.2
V3	12.1±0.4	13.8±1.1	14.1±0.7
V4	7.3±0.2	7.9±0.4	6.9±0.3

Diameters of terminal arterioles (A4), confluent venules (V4) and vessels supplying and/or draining them (A3 and V3) in control and stimulated extensor digitorum muscle. Values in μm; means±SEM.
*$p<0.05$ versus control

growth factor (FGF-2), which could be released from it, does not seem to be involved (Brown et al. 1998). In contrast, mRNA for VEGF doubled after only 1 day of stimulation (Skorjanc et al. 1998), increased sixfold in muscles stimulated for 4 days (Hang et al. 1995), and then gradually decreased, with another peak occurring after approximately 21 days (Skorjanc et al. 1998). VEGF protein was increased after 3, 21, and 56 days of stimulation (Annex et al. 1998). Immunohistochemistry revealed a higher proportion of capillaries stained with antibodies for VEGF in muscles stimulated for 4 days (but not 2 or 3 days) than in muscles of control animals (Jeal et al. 1997). Muscle stimulation also activated another growth factor, the endothelial cell stimulating angiogenic factor (ESAF) (Brown et al. 1995a), which is known to induce endothelial cell growth in cultures and occurs in tissues with capillary growth resulting from pathological changes such as rheumatoid arthritis or diabetes (Odedra and Weiss 1991).

Thus, capillary growth in muscles whose activity was increased by chronic electrical stimulation for 8 h per day resulted in capillary proliferation within 2 days, breakage of the basement membrane after 4 days, and increased levels of mRNA for VEGF and VEGF protein, and ESAF. This could be explained by increased shear stress and possibly increased capillary wall tension. The release of prostaglandins or NO due to increased shear stress may be directly involved in capillary proliferation.

To what extent similar events can explain capillary growth in muscles exposed to long-term increases in activity by exercise training is still open to investigation. There is little doubt about the involvement of

VEGF. Circumstantial evidence indicates a possible role of blood flow as a causative factor in the initiation of capillary growth, but there are no data on microcirculation changes which would corroborate or refute the hypothesis about the role of shear stress and/or capillary wall tension in the initiation of capillary proliferation. However, Sun et al. (1994) described changes in arterioles isolated from rat gracilis muscles trained by exercise for only 2–4 weeks that could be explained by increased activity of NO synthase. This would indicate that NO may also play a role in vascular growth in endurance training.

6.4 Growth of Arterioles and Large Vessels in Skeletal Muscles Exposed to High Activity

To what extent does exercise or chronic stimulation affect growth of other branches of the vascular tree? Figure 1 demonstrates changes in capillaries, arterioles, and the whole vascular bed resulting from endurance training, albeit not in the same muscle groups. Lash and Bohlen (1992) described increased arteriolar density in the spinotrapezius muscles in rats trained by endurance training which was not accompanied by higher capillary:fiber ratio, while gracilis muscle in the same animals showed higher capillary but not arteriolar supply. In further studies, Lash (1994) found no change in resting diameters of first, second, and third order arterioles; but dilation in contracting muscles was greater in vessels wider than 30 μm than in arterioles of comparable size in untrained animals. If a similar situation occurs in humans, this might help to explain the higher maximal conductance described by Sinoway et al. (1987) and Snell et al. (1987) in the muscles of trained athletes.

The data on arteriolar and whole vascular bed growth in stimulated muscles are more conclusive. Adair et al. (1995) found doubled density in 20 μm arterioles of muscles stimulated for 52 days, with a twofold increase in the volume of the lumen in both arteries and veins. Hansen-Smith et al. (1998) followed changes in arteriolar density during early stages of stimulation, at 2 and 7 days. Arteriolar density was similar in control muscles and those stimulated for 2 days. After 7 days of stimulation, the increase was minimal in arterioles >20 μm and in the category of vessels judged as mature according to the presence of myosin heavy chains in their walls. However, there was a great increase in the

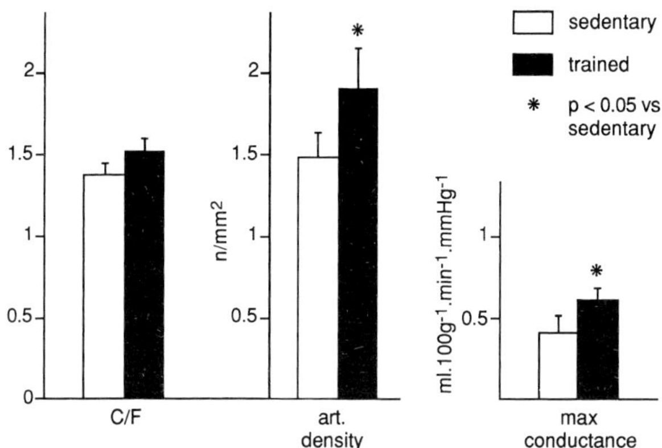

Fig. 1. Vascular bed in skeletal muscles in endurance-trained rats. Based on data from Lash and Bohlen (1992) for capillary/fiber ratio and arteriolar density in spinotrapezius muscle, and from Sexton and Laughlin (1994) for maximal conductance in hind limb muscles

number of small vessels (10 μm) stained for α smooth muscle actin (αSMA), and particularly those not completely encircled by αSMA, indicating a transformation of capillaries into arterioles, as suggested by Price et al. (1994) in developing muscles. Maximal conductance was increased in muscles stimulated for 14 days (Brown and Hudlická 1995) (Fig. 2), but probably not earlier than that, since blood flow in contracting muscles was only marginally higher after 7 days of stimulation than in control muscles (Egginton and Hudlická 1999).

It is not clear which stimulus induces growth of arterioles. Hester and Duling (1988) found only a very small increase in Vrbc in arterioles of contracting muscles, while their diameters were larger. Thus, calculated shear stress was lower rather than higher (Fig. 3). In contrast, wider diameters would result in increased circumferential wall stress, which has been shown to be an important factor in initiating arteriolar growth (Price and Skalak 1994). Therefore, it is very probable that the mechanical stimuli for capillary and arteriolar growth are different. Shear stress is an important stimulus in capillaries and circumferential wall stress in arterioles. While capillaries in stimulated muscles grow by sprouting (Myrhage and Hudlická 1978) and/or longitudinal splitting (Hansen-

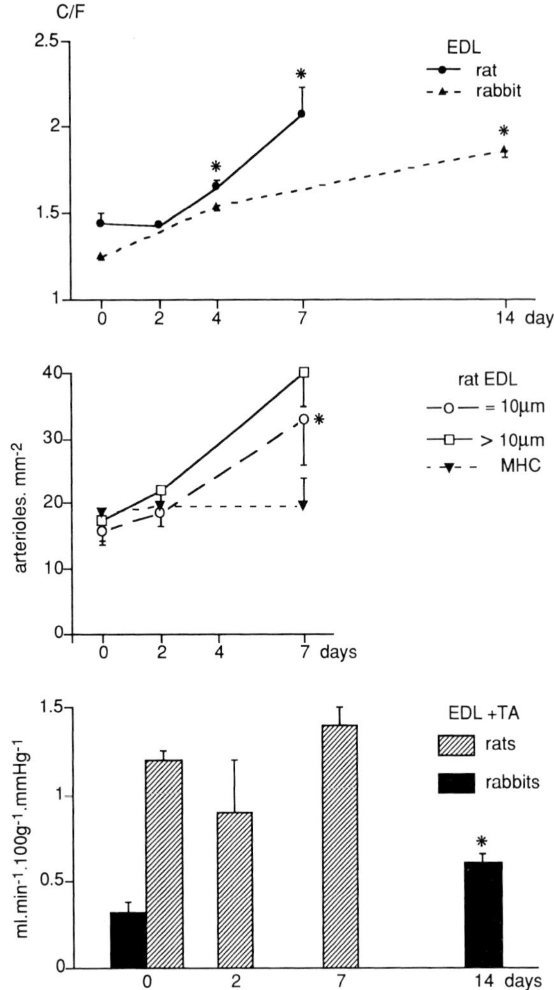

Fig. 2. Vascular bed in control (day 0) and muscles chronically stimulated for 8 h/day for up to 14 days in rats and rabbits. C:F and arteriolar density in EDL, maximal conductance in TA and EDL. *Asterisks* denote values significantly different from controls ($p<0.05$). *MHC*, arterioles stained for myosin heavy chains (presumably mature arterioles)

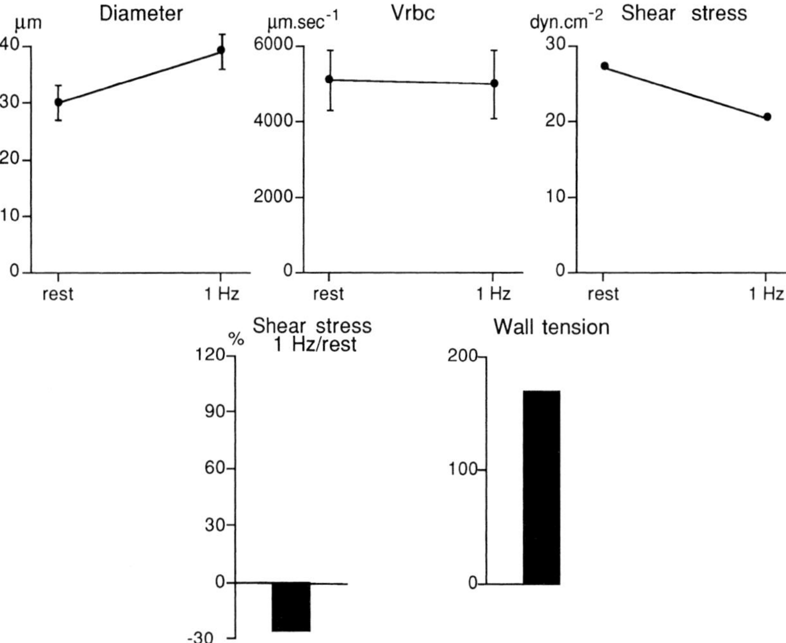

Fig. 3. Diameter, Vrbc and calculated shear stress and wall tension in arterioles at rest and during contractions at 1 Hz. Percentage change in shear stress and wall tension in contracting muscles shown in *black*. (Based on data from Hester and Duling 1988)

Smith et al. 1996), Skalak and Price (1996) suggested three possible explanations for arteriole growth. According to their scheme (Fig. 4), so-called capillary arteriolarization can occur either by migration of smooth muscle cells toward capillaries, by pericytes changing into smooth muscle cells, or by fibroblasts migrating toward capillaries and changing into smooth muscle cells.

So far, there is some support for the role of fibroblasts. Zhou and Egginton (1998) described a close apposition of proliferating fibroblasts to capillary endothelial cells in stimulated muscles using immunogold labeling for BrdU. The great increase in numbers of capillaries partially encircled by αSMA indicates either the migration of smooth muscle

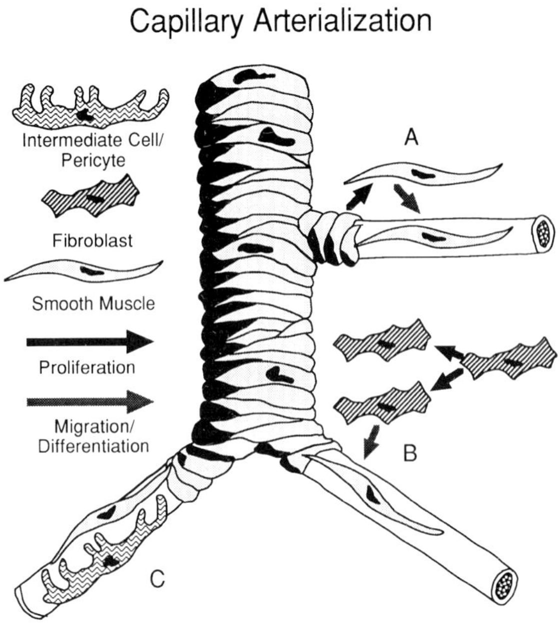

Fig. 4A–C. Schematic representation of three possible means of capillary changes into arterioles. **A** 'Arteriolarization' of capillaries by migrating vascular smooth muscle cells from arterioles towards capillaries. **B** Formation of smooth muscle cells from fibroblasts and (**C**) from pericytes. (From Skalak and Price 1996, by permission of the authors and Stockton Press)

cells or increased coverage by pericytes. However, electron microscopic studies (Egginton et al. 1996) demonstrated pericyte withdrawal, not increased coverage of the capillary circumference. So this option needs to be further examined. It remains to be seen whether the explanation of arteriolar growth in stimulated muscles can also be applied to muscles exposed to training.

To what extent the higher maximal conductance of endurance-trained and long-term stimulated muscles is a function of the increased number of arterioles, their greater capacity for dilation or enlargement of arteries is not clear. Adair et al. (1995) found that volume density of all arteries in chronically stimulated muscles increases, indicating that expansion of the vascular bed affects all vessels, not only capillaries and arterioles. This may be explained by increased eNOS activity, which was described by Delp and Laughlin (1997) in the aorta and in arterioles of exercise-trained rats by Sun et al. (1994). Thus, exercise training may cause a generalized increase of NO production and greater dilation of different vessel categories, which in turn could result in a permanent increase in vessel wall diameters and circumferential wall stress.

6.5 Effect of Training on the Vascular Bed in the Heart

It has been well-established that the hearts of so-called athletic animals (hare, wild rat) have higher capillary density (CD) than analogous, more sedentary species with similar body weights (rabbit, laboratory rats, Wachtlová et al. 1965, 1967). Flying birds have higher CD than both of the previous groups (Rakusan et al. 1971; Michel et al. 1972). Thus, it could be expected that exercise, particularly if performed vigorously for a long time, would result in an increase in CD. Surprisingly, this happens only to a limited extent, mostly in young animals.

Tomanek (1970) described increased CD in young but not adult rats trained by running. Anversa et al. (1983) found increased total capillary length under similar experimental conditions. This was later confirmed by Jacobs et al. (1984) and Mattfeldt et al. (1986), who reported increased CD as well as C:F. Capillary proliferation was demonstrated by incorporation of [^{3}H]thymidine into the nuclei of endothelial cells in the heart using electron microscopy with autoradiography (Mandache et al. 1973). Unge et al. (1979) showed it in young and adult but not old rats trained by swimming. Laughlin and McAllister (1992) concluded that capillary growth is more easily elicited by swimming than treadmill running. In cats, weight lifting had no effect at all on the size of the vascular bed (Ho et al. 1983).

Thus, capillary growth is dependent on age, type of training, and possibly species. However, it may also be related to intensity of training, although the data are controversial. Tharp and Wagner (1982) demonstrated lower CD and C:F and Anversa et al. (1982) lower capillary luminal volume density in vigorously trained rats. Vigorous training on treadmill resulted in decreased CD and total capillary length in pigs (Breisch et al. 1986), whereas it lowered CD slightly but not significantly in dogs (Laughlin and Tomanek 1987). In contrast, Leon and Bloor (1968) found an increased C:F ratio in young rats that swam for 1 h daily for 10 weeks, but not in animals trained only twice a week. When the work load was increased by carrying weights, C:F ratio increases were higher even in rats that swam only twice weekly (Bell and Rasmussen 1974).

The lack of change in capillary density does not necessarily indicate complete lack of capillary growth, since training results in mild heart hypertrophy and thus larger fibers. Therefore, unchanged CD after training implies that some capillary growth must occur, otherwise CD would decrease, as described in pathological heart hypertrophy. White et al. (1998) observed a transient increase in capillary density and [3H]thymidine labelling after 1–3 weeks of training in pig hearts but no difference from controls after 16 weeks. It is possible that a relative lack of capillary growth is due to the presence of high capillary density, since a similar lack of capillary growth was described in skeletal muscles of species with high capillary supply, such as greyhounds (see Hudlická et al. 1992).

In contrast to the controversial findings on capillary growth in animals trained by running, this exercise did increase arteriole density in pigs (Breisch et al. 1986; White et al. 1987) and rats (Rakusan and Wicker 1990). In pigs, the increase was time-dependent, with the number of smaller arterioles (10–20 μm) increasing after 8 weeks of training and in larger ones (20–30 μm) after 16 weeks (White and Bloor 1995). As there was no increase in capillary density at 8 and 16 weeks, they (White et al. 1998) proposed that the new arterioles could have arisen by transformation from capillaries, a process described in developing skeletal muscles (Price et al. 1994) that possibly also occurs in stimulated muscles (Hansen-Smith et al. 1998).

Training by running also resulted in wider diameters of large coronary arteries in humans (Froelicher 1972), dogs (Wyatt and Mitchell 1978), and rats (Thomas 1985) (Fig. 5). An increase in size of the whole coronary bed was shown by vascular casts (Tepperman and Pearlman 1961; Ho et al. 1983) and higher maximal coronary conductance (Laughlin and McAllister 1992). The latter could be due to a greater vasodilator capacity of coronary resistance arteries (Muller et al. 1994), which is endothelium-dependent (Oltman et al. 1995). This can be explained by an increase in mRNA for eNOS (Woodman et al. 1997)

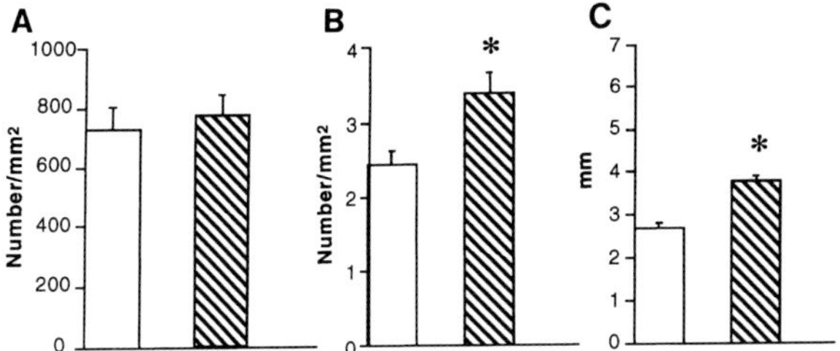

Fig. 5. Size of the vascular bed in the hearts of trained animals. Capillary density (**A**) and diameter of circumflex coronary artery (**C**) are based on the data from Wyatt and Mitchell (1978) in dogs; arteriolar density (**B**) in pigs (Breisch et al. 1986). Values from sedentary animals are represented by empty columns, in endurance-trained animals by hatched columns. *Asterisk* denotes values significantly different from sedentary animals ($p<0.05$)

and could result in remodeling of the coronary vascular bed. White and Bloor (1995) found that an increase in the number of vessels accounted for only an 11% increase in the size of the coronary vascular bed in trained pigs, while the cross sectional area increased by 50%.

6.6 Hemodynamic and Mechanical Factors Involved in the Growth of the Coronary Vascular Bed

It is well known that coronary blood flow increases with each bout of dynamic exercise, and it is possible that mechanical factors acting on the vessel walls (such as shear stress or wall tension), coupled with increased blood flow, may stimulate vessel growth, either by enlargement of the diameter (in the case of large arteries) or by an increase in the number of branches (in the case of arterioles and/or capillaries). Training also results in long-term bradycardia with longer periods of flow during prolonged diastole and increased capillary wall tension, since capillary diameters are larger during diastole than during systole (Tillmanns et al. 1974). In addition, training has a positive inotropic effect, and increased force of contraction may affect the extracellular matrix and the deformation of blood vessels, particularly capillaries (Hudlická et al. 1995).

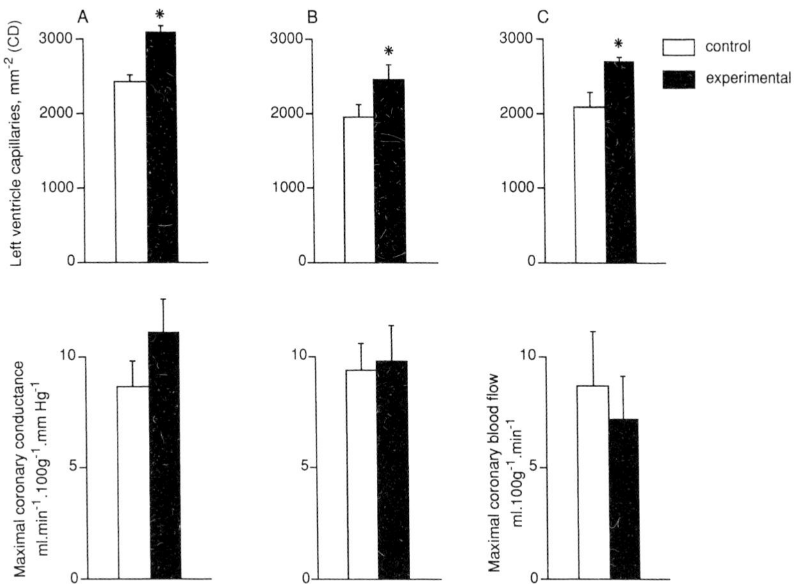

Fig. 6A–C. Capillary density and maximal coronary conductance in rabbits. **A** Animals treated for 3–5 weeks by IV infusion of adenosine (or saline) (data from Ziada et al. 1984). **B** Animals bradycardially paced for 4 weeks (data from Wright and Hudlická 1981; Hudlická et al. 1989). **C** Animals treated for 2 weeks by IV infusion of dobutamine(or saline) (data from Brown and Hudlická 1991). *Asterisks* denote values significantly different from controls ($p<0.05$)

Ziada et al. (1984) found increased capillary density without any changes in maximal coronary conductance (Fig. 6A) in the hearts of rabbits who received adenosine or propentofylline for 3–5 weeks by continuous IV infusion; neither heart rate nor stroke work were altered. Other investigators achieved capillary proliferation by long-term administration of dipyridamole (Tornling et al. 1978) or alcohol (Mall et al. 1982; for review see Hudlická and Brown 1996). The specificity of increased blood flow on capillary growth has been demonstrated in experiments with administration of α1 blocker prazosin. This drug trebled flow in skeletal muscle but did not alter it in the heart and, after a 5-week administration, increased capillary supply in the former but

Table 3. Shear stress and wall tension in capillaries in paced hearts

	Systole Control	Paced	Diastole Control	Paced
Duration (s)	0.12	0.22	0.16	0.28
Diameter (μm)	4.1±0.6		6.3±0.6	
Vrbc (μm/s)	315±60		143±90	
Assumed cap (P)	12 mmHg			
Shear stress dyne.cm^{-2}	123		36	
Wall tension dyne.cm^{-1}	24.6		37.8	

Calculated capillary shear stress and capillary wall tension in systole and diastole in control and bradycardially paced hearts. Heart rate in conscious control rabbits was 217, in paced animals, 120 beats per minute. (values for diameters, vrbc and P from Tillmanns et al. 1974; Nellis and Liedtke 1982)

not in the latter (Ziada et al. 1989). Vasodilators elevate capillary Vrbc without affecting their diameters (Tillmanns et al. 1982) and thus increase wall shear stress (Hudlická 1994), which could stimulate capillary growth by mechanisms discussed above in connection with capillary growth in chronically stimulated muscles.

Prolonged bradycardia may be another factor stimulating capillary growth. Since capillary diameters are larger during diastole than systole, although their pressures do not seem to be different, capillary wall tension increases (Hudlická et al. 1995, Table 3). During bradycardia, this occurs for relatively long periods of time. This may cause disruption of the capillary basement membrane and enable endothelial cell migration and consecutive capillary elongation.

The relationship between heart rate and capillary supply has been demonstrated with both lower and higher heart rates: Poupa et al. (1970) showed that higher capillary density in “athletic” animals is linked to lower heart rates, while Mattfeldt and Mall (1987) found lower capillary density and total capillary length in animals with higher heart rates. Rapid atrial pacing for 3 weeks also decreased the total volume density of capillaries (Spinale et al. 1992). Heart rate reduction by alinidine (Schamhardt et al. 1981) or acute bradycardial pacing (Indolfi et al. 1991) improved subendocardial perfusion in ischemic hearts and, if a similar effect occurs in normal hearts, bradycardia may increase both wall shear stress and capillary wall tension. Whatever the mechanism of resting bradycardia in response to training, it was an effective promoter of capillary growth only in young animals. It could be that a much more drastic reduction in heart rate is needed to induce capillary growth in adults. With this in mind, we attempted to stimulate capillary growth by a drastic reduction in heart rate achieved either by electrical bradycardial pacing in rabbits (Wright and Hudlická 1981) and pigs (Brown et al. 1994), or by long-term administration of alinidine, a drug with predominantly negative chronotropic effects, in rats (Brown et al. 1990). An increase in capillary density was demonstrated after 3–4 weeks of pacing, estimated on the basis of histochemical staining of vessels for alkaline phosphatase (rabbits and rats), by binding of the lectin Griffonia simplicifolia I (pigs), or by low-power electron microscopy, and was found to occur in the absence of changes in myocyte diameters.

The greater the bradycardia, the greater the increase in capillary density. Heart rate reduction by about 50% in rabbits resulted in almost 30% higher capillary density than in the animals with a comparable heart weight, while the 30% reduction in pigs and rats was linked with 20% higher CD (Hudlická and Brown 1996). In contrast to endurance training, there was no change in the maximal coronary conductance (Fig. 6B), thus indicating that bradycardia stimulated growth of capillaries without accompanying growth of larger vessels. Although the coronary flow per beat was higher (Hudlická et al. 1989), it is unlikely that increased shear stress could explain capillary growth, since Vrbc is much higher during systole than during diastole and the relative duration of systole is not dramatically shortened even with a drastic reduction in heart rate. However, since capillaries are wider during diastole, the calculated capillary wall tension would be considerably higher in bradycardially paced rabbit hearts than the control ones (Table 3).

Yet another mechanical stimulus for vessel growth resulting from endurance training may be linked to mechanical distortion of the heart from either elongation of myocytes during prolonged diastole or increased contraction force due to positive inotropism. Since capillaries are tethered to myocytes, exaggerated changes in myocyte contraction could result in a disturbance of their basement membrane and/or extracellular matrix and initiate the angiogenesis cascade with endothelial cell migration and proliferation. The importance of the latter factor in initiating capillary growth could be determined by studying the effect of drugs with positive inotropic action.

Long-term administration of a beta agonist dobutamine increased the stroke volume with a concomitant decrease in coronary blood flow in dogs (Liang et al. 1979) and simulated some effects of training in rats (Buttrick et al. 1988). In rabbits, it had a positive inotropic and minimal chronotropic effect when given by continuous IV infusion for 2 weeks. It did not cause heart hypertrophy but increased maximal stroke work and capillary density without affecting maximal coronary blood flow (Fig. 6C), thus demonstrating an effect on growth of capillaries but not of larger vessels (Brown and Hudlická 1991).

When all three components of the endurance training – increased coronary blood flow, long-term bradycardia, and positive inotropic effect – are studied separately, it is obvious that each can induce capillary growth but does not increase maximal coronary conductance, a result contrary to that seen in endurance training. This discrepancy may be explained by the fact that endurance training results in a relatively smaller changes in resting heart rate, coronary flow, and increased inotropism than those experimentally induced to an exaggerated degree with vasodilators, bradycardia, or dobutamine. It is also possible that a combination of all three components has a different effect than each procedure applied on its own. Furthermore, vascular bed changes in endurance-trained animals and humans were studied after a much longer period of time, and it is possible that after several weeks of training, in contrast to the days used in other experimental protocols, capillaries had already been transformed into arterioles by a process similar to that described in skeletal muscles and recently confirmed in pig hearts (White et al. 1998).

Mechanical factors resulting from changes in blood flow, heart rate, elongation of myocytes during prolonged diastole, or increased force of contraction could also lead to activation of growth factors. Zheng and Tomanek (1998) found increased levels of mRNA for VEGF in rat hearts with bradycardia elicited by administration of alinidine; and Hudlická et al. (1995) showed a good correlation between capillary density and levels of ESAF in bradycardially paced hearts, while mRNA for FGF-2 did not seem to be related to capillary supply.

6.7 Effect of Altered Hemodynamic Factors on Growth of Vessels in Ischemic Muscles

Reports on the occurrence of angiogenesis in ischemic muscles are very controversial. It could be assumed that limitation of blood supply would result in loss of capillaries, but only Clyne et al. (1985) described decreased capillary supply in muscles of patients suffering from peripheral vascular diseases, while others (e.g., Hammarsten et al. 1980; Henriksson et al. 1980; Jansson et al. 1988; Esbjornsson et al. 1993) found no change. Since the resting blood flow is usually not impaired, maintenance of minimal perfusion obviously contributes to the preservation of the integrity of the capillary bed. This has been shown in animal experiments where ligation of the common iliac artery did not result in any loss of capillaries 7–35 days later, although the volume flow per capillary was slightly lower (Dawson and Hudlická 1990). However, since Vrbc was increased, shear stress in individual capillaries was not lower than in control muscles (Hudlická et al. 1998b). This could help to prevent capillary loss by maintaining NO release. Muronara et al. (1998) described loss of capillaries in eNOS-deficient mice with ligated femoral arteries, while capillary growth was enhanced in ischemic muscles in l-arginine-fed rabbits.

Proliferation of capillaries was also reported 1 week after ligation of the femoral artery, but only in muscles with a high proportion of glycolytic fibers (gastrocnemius). This was attributed to hypoxia, while extensive development of larger vessels in the thigh was explained partly by dilation of existing vessels, and partly by proliferation of endothelial cells and smooth muscle cells in their vessel wall (Ito et al. 1997).

Growth of larger vessels and capillaries was previously demonstrated by increased incorporation of [^{3}H]thymidine in dog calf muscles after surgical popliteal arteriovenous anastomosis (Sewell and Roth 1958) and by direct observation of the numbers of small arterioles in rat cremaster muscle 3 weeks after ligation of the main feeding vessel (Hogan and Hirschman 1984).

Whether hemodynamic factors can explain such extensive vascular remodeling and growth in skeletal muscle vasculature in situations of decreased blood flow is still open to speculation. It has been suggested that decreased pressure below the site of an obstruction would result in

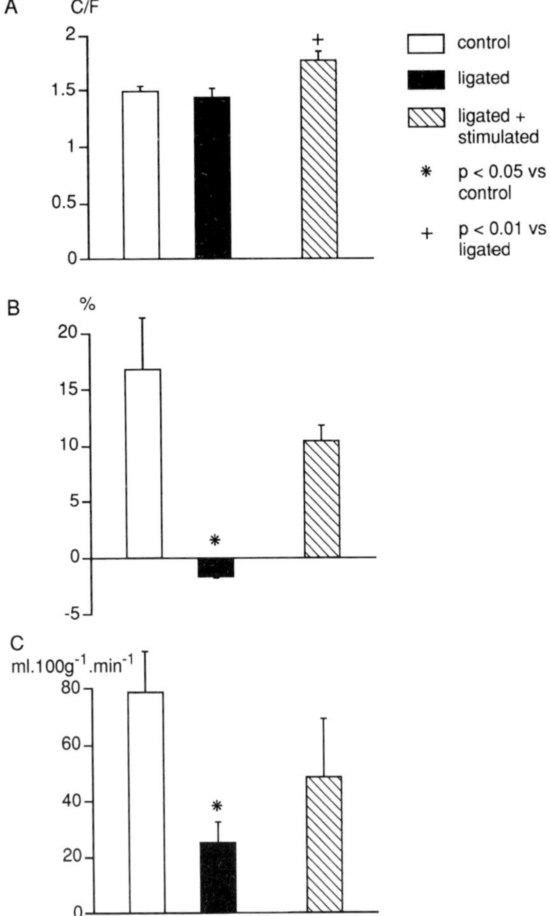

Fig. 7A–C. Changes in the vascular bed in rat control, ischemic and ischemic-stimulated ankle flexors 2 weeks after ligation of the common iliac artery. **A** Capillary/fiber (C:F) ratio in EDL. **B** Percent increase in diameters in terminal arterioles (*A4*) in TA during contraction at 1 Hz. **C** Maximal blood flow measured by microspheres in contracting TA and EDL. (Based on data from Hudlická et al. 1994)

dilation and increased wall tension (John and Warren 1961) while Ito et al. (1997) suggested that increased maximal collateral conductance possibly due to changed reactivity of arterioles may increase shear stress and upregulate growth factors in the vessel wall.

Can exercise training or vasodilating drugs enhance development of collateral circulation? Although exercise is the most successful therapy for peripheral vascular diseases (reviewed by Regensteiner 1997), more recent studies did not report increases in overall muscle blood flow. However, earlier studies (e.g., Zetterquist 1970) showed improved nutritive muscle flow in calf muscles in humans. This could explain the increased C:F ratio described by Yang et al. (1991) in ankle extensors in rats with limited blood supply trained by running, in spite of the previous reports that training did not improve collateral development (Sanne and Sivertsson 1968; Mathien and Terjung 1986, 1990; Roberts et al. 1997).

However, blood flow increases with every muscle contraction and, even if this increase is much smaller than in muscles with unlimited blood supply (Hughes and Hudlická 1992), the increased capillary shear stress can contribute to increased capillarization by mechanisms described above. Increased blood flow by long-term administration of $\alpha 1$ antagonist prazosin (which was found to increase capillary shear stress in normal muscles; Dawson and Hudlická 1993) also induced capillary growth and improved muscle blood flow and performance in ischemic muscles (Fulgenzi et al. 1998).

A more specific increase in muscle activity induced by chronic electrical stimulation applied for 10–15 min seven times per day for 2 weeks improved muscle blood flow, restored the ability of arterioles to dilate (which was impaired in ischemic muscles, Dawson et al. 1990), and stimulated capillary growth (Fig. 7). It also increased perfusion pressure below the site of ligation, indicating inflow from either preexisting or newly grown collaterals (Hudlická et al. 1994). Thus, shear stress may play an important role in the maintenance of capillary integrity in ischemic muscles and in capillary growth induced by increased muscle activity or long-term use of vasodilators. Although we have so far no data on the effect of chronic electrical stimulation on capillary growth in ischemic muscles in man, it improved significantly muscle performance in patients with intermittent claudication (Tsang et al. 1994).

6.8 Are Hemodynamic Factors Involved in Angiogenesis in the Ischemic Heart?

Some angiogenesis occurs in ischemic hearts without any intervention. An increase in arteriolar density and some capillary sprouting were observed 2–5 days after partial constriction of the coronary artery (White et al. 1990). Recent reports (Shammas et al. 1993; Xie et al. 1997) describe angiogenesis in tissue close to the infarct attributable to the presence of either thrombin, a potent angiogenic factor, or other growth factors rather than to hemodynamic changes. However, hearts with limited blood supply usually show a deficit in capillaries (Anversa et al. 1986), but this is mainly due to hypertrophy of the remaining viable tissue.

It is extremely difficult, particularly in the heart, to measure in vivo relevant parameters such as flow velocity and vessel diameter from which the involvement of hemodynamic factors could be calculated. Tillmanns et al. (1974, 1981, 1982) measured diameter and pressure in epicardial arterioles and venules, and diameters and red blood cell velocities of capillaries in normal hearts from different species, but not during development of collateral circulation. Schaper (1971) considered tangential shear stress (t=PR/D, where D =wall thickness, P=pressure, and R=radius) an important factor in the development of collaterals in the heart, assuming that hypoxia rather than pressure gradient was the main cause of vessel dilation.

The dilator role of hypoxia was also confirmed in studies showing better collateral development in patients experiencing angina (Schaper et al. 1981) or after ischemic preconditioning (i.e., repeated, short-duration coronary artery occlusions) (Sasayama and Fujita 1992; Tomoike 1993). Kern et al. (1993) found about 30% higher velocity of flow in patients with a partially or fully occluded coronary artery distal to the occlusion, but there are no comparable data on the diameters of these vessels from which relative change in shear stress could be calculated. Ware and Simons (1997) suggest that formation of collaterals is enhanced by shear stress and growth factors in the areas around the occlusion of larger arteries, but that angiogenesis in the distal ischemic zones is helped mainly by inflammation and the presence of neutrophils and macrophages which may release various growth factors.

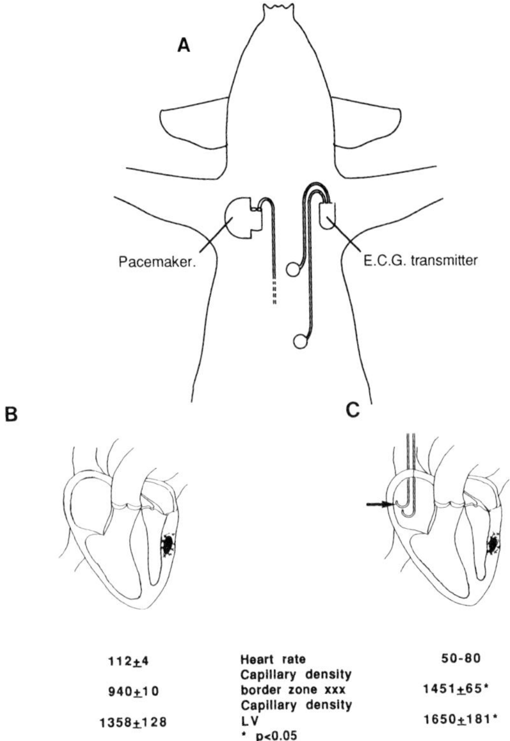

Fig. 8. Changes in capillary density in infarcted and infarcted bradycardially paced pig hearts. **A** Scheme of bradycardial pacing in pigs (Brown et al. 1994). Scheme of infarction with values for heart rate, capillary density in the border zone to infarction and in the intact left ventricle in infarcted pigs (**B**) and in infarcted bradycardially paced pigs (**C**). *Arrow* indicates the position of pacing electrodes (based on data from Brown et al. 1995b). Infarct marked in black

The question of whether development of collateral circulation can be enhanced by interventions such as exercise training or drugs is still unanswered (for reviews see Hudlická et al. 1992; Tomanek 1994). Although recent data show that only very vigorous training can protect against coronary heart disease (Morris 1994), mortality in patients with nonfatal myocardial infarction has dropped, possibly because exercise slows the progression of arteriosclerosis and leads to adaptations in skeletal muscles, which reduce demands on cardiac output rather than improving blood supply to the heart (Chandrasherkhar and Anand 1991; McKirnan and Bloor 1994; Libonati et al. 1997).

In contrast, exercise may stimulate vessel growth in animals. Exercise-trained rats had higher blood flow in the border zone to the ischemic area after ligation of the coronary artery, which could explain the normalization of the C:F ratios in this zone (Przyklenk and Groom 1984, 1985). Bloor et al. (1984) found that exercise training in pigs also increased collateral flow primarily in the vicinity of the ischemic area. Heaton et al. (1978) explained improved flow close to the infarcted areas in trained dogs as a consequence of training-induced bradycardia. Bradycardia generated by pacing (Brown et al. 1994) shortly after occlusion of the left descending coronary artery and maintained for 4 weeks resulted in considerably higher capillary density in the border zone as well as in the part of left ventricle unaffected by infarction when compared with infarcted hearts, whose heart rate was not altered by any intervention (Brown et al. 1995b) (Fig. 8).

As mentioned above, bradycardia may help stimulate capillary growth by increased capillary wall tension and possible release of growth factors, and it certainly would be important to explore its further use in capillary growth in infarcted hearts. Indeed, drugs which lower heart rate increased flow in collaterals when administered acutely to dogs with myocardial infarction (Daemmgen and Gross 1985; Gross and Daemmgen 1987). However, zatebradine, which lowered heart rates by 20% in patients with angina both at rest and during exercise, did not increase the length of time that patients were able to exercise (Glaser 1997). Presently, it is impossible to establish whether this difference is due to a different effect of bradycardic drugs in animals and in humans – similar to the effect of exercise on the development of collateral circulation – or to different conditions (infarction compared with a stable angina).

Conclusions

Endurance training results in an increased size of the capillary and possibly whole vascular bed in skeletal muscles, which might be partly explained by hemodynamic factors, upregulation of NO synthase, and a greater capacity of arterioles to dilate. However, precise evidence on the roles of shear stress or circumferential wall stress in vascular bed growth in exercise-trained muscles is not yet available. Intensive increases in activity by electrical stimulation of small muscle groups induced capillary proliferation within only 2 days, growth of arterioles within 7 days, and increase in the size of the whole vascular bed between 7 and 14 days.

Increased shear stress, and consequent release of NO and prostaglandins play a crucial role in growth of capillaries, while increased wall tension (circumferential wall stress) is an important factor in growth of arterioles. In the heart, training rarely results in capillary growth, but induces growth of arterioles and expansion of conduit arteries. In contrast, a long-term increase in blood flow by various vasodilators, long-term bradycardia, or increased inotropism (by β-agonist dobutamine) all induced capillary growth without changes in the maximal coronary conductance, indicating that the size of the whole coronary vascular bed was not altered.

Exercise stimulates growth of collaterals in ischemic skeletal and cardiac muscles in animals, but there is little proof that it can enhance it in man (Firoozan and Forfar 1996). Chronic electrical stimulation induced growth of capillaries in ischemic muscles in animals and improved muscle performance in patients, and long-term bradycardia stimulated growth of capillaries in the border zone to infarction. However, its possible use in man has to be explored.

References

Adair TH, Hang J, Wells ML, McGee FD, Montani JP (1995) Long-term electrical stimulation of rabbit skeletal muscle increases growth of paired arteries and veins. Am J Physiol 38:H717–724

Andersen P, Henriksson J (1977) Capillary supply of the quadriceps femoris muscle of man: adaptive response to exercise. J Physiol (Lond) 270:677–690

Ando J, Nomura H, Kamyia A (1987) The effect of fluid shear stress on the migration and proliferation of cultured endothelial cells. Microvasc Res 33:62–70

Annex BH, Torgan CE, Lin P, Taylor DA, Thompson MA, Peters KG, Kraus WE (1998) Induction and maintenance of increased VEGF protein by chronic motor nerve stimulation in skeletal muscle. Am J Physiol 274:H860–867

Anversa P, Beghi PC, Levicky V, McDonald SL, Kikkawa Y (1982) Morphometry of right ventricular hypertrophy induced by strenuous exercise in rat. Am J Physiol 243:H850–861

Anversa P, Levicky V, Beghi C, McDonald SL, Kikkawa Y (1983) Morphometry of exercise-induced right ventricular hypertrophy in the rat. Circ Res 52:57–64

Anversa P, Beghi C, Kikkawa Y,Olivetti G (1986) Myocardial infarction in rats. Infarct size, myocyte hypertrophy and capillary growth. Circ Res 58:26–37

Armstrong RB, Laughlin MH (1983) Blood flows within and among rat muscles as a function of time during high speed treadmill exercise. J Physiol (Lond) 344:189–208

Bell RD, Rasmussen RL (1974) Exercise and the myocardial capillary-fiber ratio during growth. Growth 38:237–244

Ben Ezra D (1978) Neovasculogenic ability of prostaglandins,growth factors and synthetic chemoattractants. Am J Ophthalmol 86:455–461

Bloor CM, White FC, Sanders TM (1984) Effects of exercise on collateral development in myocardial ischemia in pigs. J Appl Physiol 56:656–665

Breen EC, Johnson EC, Wagner H, Tseng HM, Sung LA, Wagner PD (1996) Angiogenic growth factor mRNA responses in muscle to a single bout of exercise. J Appl Physiol 81:355–361

Breisch EA, White FC, Nimmo LE, McKirnan MD, Bloor CM (1986) Exercise-induced cardiac hypertrophy, a correlation of blood flow and microvasculature. J Appl Physiol 60:1259–1267

Brown MD, Hudlická O (1991) Capillary supply and cardiac performance in the rabbit after chronic dobutamine treatment. Cardiovasc Res 25:909–915

Brown MD, Hudlická O (1995) Vascular conductance and capillary supply in heart and skeletal muscle in response to altered activity. Microcirculation 2:98

Brown MD, Cotter M, Hudlická O, Vrbova G (1976) The effect of different patterns of muscle activity on capillary density, mechanical properties and structure of slow and fast rabbit muscles. Pflugers Arch 361:241–250

Brown MD, Cleasby MJ, Hudlická O (1990) Capillary supply of hypertrophied rat hearts after chronic treatment with the bradycardic agent alinidine. J Physiol (Lond) 427:40P

Brown MD, Davies MK, Hudlická O, Townsend P (1994) Long-term bradycardia by electrical pacing: a new method for studying heart rate reduction. Cardiovasc Res 28:1774–1779

Brown MD, Hudlická O, Makki RF, Weiss JB (1995a) Low-molecular-mass endothelial cell-stimulating angiogenic factor in relation to capillary growth induced in rat skeletal muscle by low-frequency electrical stimulation. Int J Microcirc 15:111–116

Brown MD, Davies M, Hudlická O, Townsend P (1995b) Capillary density and performance in bradycardially paced infarcted pig hearts. J Mol Cell Cardiol 27:A91

Brown MD, Walter HJ, Hansen-Smith FM, Hudlická O, Egginton S (1998) Lack of involvement of basic fibroblast growth factor (FGF-2) in capillary growth in skeletal muscles exposed to long-term contractile activity. Angiogenesis 2:81–21

Buttrick PM, Malhotra A, Factor S, Greenen D, Scheuer J (1988) Effect of chronic dobutamine administration on hearts of normal and hypertensive rats. Circ Res 63:173–181

Chandrasherkhar Y, Anand IS (1991) Exercise as a coronary protective factor. Am Heart J 122:1723–1739

Clyne CAC, Mears H, Weller RO, O'Donnell TF (1985) Calf muscle adaptation to peripheral vascular disease. Cardiovasc Res 19:507–512

Daemmgen JW, Gross GJ (1985) AQ-AH 208, a new bradycardic agent, increases coronary collateral blood flow to ischemic myocardium. J Cardiovasc Pharmacol 7:1048–1054

Dawson JM (1987) Responses of the microcirculation in metabolically different skeletal muscles to increased and reduced blood flow. PhD thesis, University of Birmingham

Dawson JM, Hudlická O (1989) The effect of long-term activity on the microvasculature of rat glycolytic skeletal muscle. Int J Microcirc 8:53–59

Dawson JM, Hudlická O (1990) Changes in the microcirculation in slow and fast skeletal muscles with long-term limitation of blood supply. Cardiovasc Res 24:390–395

Dawson JM, Hudlická O (1993) Can changes in microcirculation explain capillary growth in skeletal muscle? Int J Exp Pathol 74:65–71

Dawson JM, Tyler KR, Hudlická O (1987) A comparison of the microcirculation in rat fast glycolytic and slow oxidative muscles at rest and during contractions. Microvas Res 33:167–182

Dawson JM, Okyayuz-Baklouti I, Hudlická O (1990) Skeletal muscle microcirculation: the effects of limited blood supply and treatment with torbafylline. Int J Microcirc 9:385–400

Delp MM, Laughlin MH (1997) Time course of enhanced endothelium-mediated dilation in the aorta of trained rats. Med Sci Sports Exerc 29:1454–1461

Duling BR, Dejardins C (1987) Capillary hematocrit – what does it mean? NIPS 2:66–69

Egginton S, Hudlická O (1989) The effect of long-term activation of glycolytic fibers in rat skeletal muscle on capillary supply and enzyme activities. J Physiol (Lond) 409:71P

Egginton S, Hudlická O (1999) Early changes in performance, blood flow and capillary fine structure in rat fast muscles induced by electrical stimulation. J Physiol (Lond) 515:265–275

Egginton S, Hudlická O, Brown MD, Graciotti L, Granata AL (1996) In vivo pericyte-endothelial cell interaction during angiogenesis in adult cardiac and skeletal muscle. Microvasc Res 51:213–228

Esbjornsson M, Jansson E, Sundberg CJ, Sylven C, Eiken O, Nygren A, Kaijser L (1993) Muscle fiber types and enzyme activities after training with local leg ischaemia in man. Acta Physiol Scand 148:233–241

Firoozan S, Forfar JC (1996) Exercise training and the coronary collateral circulation: is its value underestimated in man? Eur Heart J 17:1791–1795

Froelicher VF (1972) Animal studies of effect of chronic exercise on the heart and atherosclerosis. Am Heart J 84:496–506

Form DH, Auerbach R (1983) PGE2 and angiogenesis. Proc Soc Exp Biol Med 172:214–218

Fulgenzi G, Graciotti L, Collis MG, Hudlická O (1998) The effect of alpha-1 adrenoceptor antagonist prazosin on capillary supply, blood flow and performance in a rat model of chronic muscle ischaemia. Eur J Vasc Endovasc Surg 16:71–77

Glaser SP (1997) Effects of zatebradine (ULFS 49CL), a sinus node inhibitor,on heart rate and exercise duration in chronic stable angina pectoris. Am J Cardiol 79:1401–1404

Gray SD, Renkin EM (1978) Microvascular supply in relation to fiber metabolic type in mixed skeletal muscle of rabbits. Microvasc Res 16:406–425

Gross GJ, Daemmgen JW (1987) Effect of the new specific bradycardial agent AQ-A39 (Falipamil) on coronary collateral blood flow in dogs. J Cardiovasc Pharmacol 10:123–127

Gute D, Laughlin MH, Amann JF (1994) Regional changes in capillary supply in skeletal muscle of interval-sprint and low-intensity, endurance-trained rats. Microcirculation 1:183–193

Gute D, Fraga C, Laughlin MH, Amann JF (1996) Regional changes in capillary supply in skeletal muscle of high-intensity endurance-trained rats. J Appl Physiol 81:619–616

Hammarsten J, Bylund-Fellenius NC, Holm J, Schersten T, Krotkiewski M (1980) Capillary supply and muscle fiber types in patients with intermittent claudication: relationship between morphology and metabolism. Eur J Clin Invest 10:301–305

Hang J, Kong L, Gu J-W, Adair TH (1995) VEGF gene expression is upregulated in electrically stimulated rat skeletal muscle. Am J Physiol 269:H1827–H1831

Hansen-Smith FM, Hudlická O, Egginton S (1996) In vivo angiogenesis in adult rat skeletal muscle: early changes in capillary network architecture and ultrastructure. Cell Tissue Res 286:123–136

Hansen-Smith FM, Egginton S, Hudlická O (1998) Growth of arterioles in chronically stimulated adult skeletal muscle. Microcirculation 5:49–59

Heaton WH, Marr KC, Capurro NL, Goldstein RE, Epstein SE (1978) Beneficial effect of physical training on blood flow to myocardium perfused by chronic collaterals in the exercising dog. Circulation 57:575–581

Henriksson J, Nygaard E, Andersson J, Eklöf B (1980) Enzyme activities, fiber types and capillarization in calf muscles of patients with intermittent claudication. Scand J Clin Lab Invest 40:361–369

Hester RL, Duling B (1988) Red cell velocity during functional hyperemia: implications for rheology and oxygen transport. Am J Physiol 255:H236–244

Ho KW, Roy RR, Taylor JF, Heusner WW, Van Huss WD (1983) Differential effects of running and weight-lifting on the rat coronary arterial tree. Med Sci Sports Exerc 15:472–477

Hogan RD, Hirschmann L (1984) Arteriolar proliferation in the rat cremaster muscle as a long-term autoregulatory response to reduced perfusion. Microvasc Res 27:290–296

Hoppeler H, Desplanches D (1992) Muscle structural modifications in hypoxia. Int J Sports Med 143 [Suppl 1]:S166–168

Hudlická O (1975) Uptake of substrates in slow and fast muscles in situ. Microvasc Res 10:17–28

Hudlická O (1991) What makes blood vessels grow? J Physiol (Lond) 444:1–24

Hudlická O (1994) Mechanical factors involved in the growth of the heart and its blood vessels. Cell Mol Biol Res 40:143–152

Hudlická O (1998) Is physiological angiogenesis in skeletal muscle regulated by changes in microcirculation? Microcirculation 5:7–23

Hudlická O, Brown MD (1993) Physical forces in angiogenesis. In: Rubanyi G (ed) Mechanoreception by the vascular wall. Futura, Mount Kisco, p 197–241

Hudlická O, Brown MD (1996) Postnatal growth of the heart and its blood vessels. J Vasc Res 33:266–287

Hudlická O, Egginton S (1994) Early changes in muscle blood flow and performance induced by chronic electrical stimulation of rat fast muscles. J Physiol (Lond) 477:37P

Hudlická O, Tyler KR (1984) The effect of long-term high frequency stimulation on capillary density and fiber types in rabbit fast muscles. J Physiol (Lond) 353:435–445

Hudlická O, Dodd L, Renkin EM, Gray SD (1982) Early changes in fiber profile and capillary density in long-term stimulated muscles. Am J Physiol 243:H528–535

Hudlická O, Tyler KR, Wright AJA, Ziada AMAR (1984) Growth of capillaries in skeletal muscles. Prog Appl Microcirc 5:44–64

Hudlická O, West D, Kumar S, El Khelly F, Wright AJA (1989) Can growth of capillaries in the heart and skeletal muscle be explained by the presence of an angiogenic factor? Br J Exp Pathol 70:237–246

Hudlická O, Brown MD, Egginton S (1992) Angiogenesis in skeletal and cardiac muscle. Physiol Rev 72:369–417

Hudlická O, Brown MD, Egginton S, Dawson JM (1994) Effect of long-term electrical stimulation on vascular supply and fatigue in chronically ischemic muscles. J Appl Physiol 77:1317–1324

Hudlická O, Brown MD, Walter H, Weiss JB, Bate A (1995) Factors involved in capillary growth in the heart. Mol Cell Biochem 147:57–68

Hudlická O, Brown MD, Silgram H (1996) Role of nitric oxide in capillary proliferation in chronically stimulated rat skeletal muscle. Int J Microcirc 16(S1):P92

Hudlická O, Brown MD, Egginton S (1998a) Angiogenesis: basic concepts and methodology. In: Halliday A, Hunt BJ, Poston L, Schachter M (eds) An introduction to vascular biology. Cambridge University Press, Cambridge, p 3–19

Hudlická O, Brown MD, Dawson JM (1998b) Growth and regression of capillaries in rabbit and rat skeletal muscles. J Physiol (Lond) 511P:158P

Hughes RA, Hudlická O (1992) Changes in capillary ultrastructure, blood flow and muscle performance during development of collateral circulation in rat fast muscles. J Physiol (Lond) 452:115P

Indolfi C, Goth B.D, Miyazaki S, Miura T, Schulz R, Ross J Jr (1991) Heart rate reduction improves myocardial ischemia in swine – role of interventricular blood flow redistribution. Am J Physiol 261:H910–917

Ingjer F (1979) Effects of endurance training on muscle fiber ATPase activity, capillary supply and mitochondrial content in man. J Physiol (Lond) 294:419–432

Ito WD, Arras M, Scholz D, Winkler B, Htun P, Schaper W (1997) Angiogenesis but not collateral growth is associated with ischemia of the femoral artery occlusion. Am J Physiol 273:H1255–1265

Jacobs TB, Bell RD, McClements JD (1984) Exercise, age and the development of the myocardial vasculature. Growth 48:148–157

Jansson E, Johansson J, Sylven C, Kaijser L (1988) Calf muscle adaptation in intermittent claudication. Clin Physiol 8:17–29

Jeal S, Brown MD, Hudlická O, Egginton S (1997) Involvement of vascular endothelial growth factor in capillary growth as a result of chronic electrical stimulation of skeletal muscle in conscious rats. J Physiol (Lond) 499:39P

John HT, Warren R (1961) The stimulus to collateral circulation. Surgery 49:14–25

Kern MJ, Donohue TJ, Bach RG, Aguirre FV, Caracciolo EA, Ofili EO (1993) Quantitating coronary collateral flow velocity in patients during coronary angioplasty using a Doppler guide wire. Am J Cardiol 71:34D–40D

Koller A, Kaley G (1996) Shear stress dependent regulation of vascular resistance in health and disease: role of endothelium. Endothelium 4:247–272

Lash JM (1994) Contribution of arterial feed vessels to skeletal muscle functional hyperemia. J Appl Physiol 76:1512–1519

Lash JM, Bohlen HG (1992) Functional adaptations of rat skeletal muscle arterioles to aerobic exercise training. J Appl Physiol 72:2052–2062

Laughlin MH, McAllister RM (1992) Exercise training-induced coronary vascular adaptation. J Appl Physiol 73:2209–2225

Laughlin MH, Armstrong RB (1982) Muscle blood flow distribution patterns as a function of running speed in rats. Am J Physiol 243:H296–306

Laughlin MH, Tomanek RJ (1987) Myocardial capillarity and maximal capillary diffusion capacity in exercise-trained dogs. J Appl Physiol 63:1481–1486

Laughlin MH, Korthuis RJ, Sexton WL, Armstrong RB (1988) Regional blood flow capacity and exercise hyperemia in high intensity trained rats. J Appl Physiol 64:2420–2427

Leon AS, Bloor CM (1968) Effects of exercise and its cessation on the heart and its blood supply. J Appl Physiol 24:485–490

Liang CS, Tuttle RR, Hood WB Jr, Gavras H (1979) Conditioning effects of chronic infusion of dobutamine. Comparison with exercise training. J Clin Invest 64:613–619

Libonati JR, Gaughan JP, Hefner CA, Gow A, Paolone AM, Houser SR (1997) Reduced ischemic and reperfusion injury following exercise training. Med Sci Sports Exerc 29:809–816

Mai JV, Edgerton VR, Barnard RJ (1970). Capillarity of red,white and intermediate muscle fibers in trained and untrained guinea pigs. Experientia 26:1222–1223

Mall G, Mattfeldt T, Rieger P, Volk B, Frolov VA (1982) Morphometric analysis of the rabbit myocardium after chronic ethanol feeding – early capillary changes. Basic Res Cardiol 77:57–67

Mandache E, Unge G, Appelgren LE, Ljungqvist A (1973) The proliferation activity of the heart tissues in various forms of experimental cardiac hypertrophy studied by electron microscope autoradiography. Virchows Arch Cell Pathol 12:112–122

Mattfeldt T, Mall G (1987)Growth of capillaries and myocardial cells in the normal rat heart. J Mol Cell Cardiol 19:1237–1246

Mattfeldt T, Krämer KL, Zeitz R, Mall G (1986) Stereology of myocardial hypertrophy induced by physical exercise. Virchows Arch Pathol Anat Histopathol 409:473–484

Mathien GM, Terjung RL (1986) Influence of training following bilateral stenosis of the femoral artery in rats. Am J Physiol 250:H1050–1059

Mathien GM, Terjung RL (1990) Muscle blood flow in trained rats with peripheral arterial insufficiency. Am J Physiol 258:H759–765

McKirnan MD, Bloor CM (1994) Clinical significance of coronary vascular adaptations to exercise training. Med Sci Sports Exerc 26:1262–1268

Mellander S, Bjornberg G (1992) Regulation of vascular smooth muscle tone and capillary pressure. NIPS 7:113–119

Michel G, Buchwald H, Schoenherr H (1972) Quantitative studies on the formation of cardiac muscle fibers and capillaries in various types of domestic and wild poultry. Anat Anz 132:382–388

Morris JN (1994) Exercise in the prevention of coronary heart disease: today's best buy in public health. Med Sci Sports Exerc 26:807–814

Muller JM, Myers PR, Laughlin MH (1994) Vasodilator responses of coronary resistance arteries of exercise-trained pigs.Circulation 89:2308–2314

Muronara T, Asahara T, Silver M, Bauters C, Masuda H, Kalka C, Kerney M,Chen D, Symes JF, Fishman MC, Huang PL, Isner JM (1998) Nitric oxide synthase modulates angiogenesis in response to tissue ischemia. J Clin Invest 101:2567–2578

Myrhage R, Hudlická O (1978) Capillary growth in chronically stimulated adult skeletal muscle as studied by intravital microscopy and histological methods in rabbits and rats. Microvasc Res 16:73–90

Nellis SH, Liedtke AL (1982) Pressure dimensions in the terminal vascular bed of the myocardium determined by a new free motion technique. In: Tillmanns H, Kubler W, Zebe H (eds) Microcirculation of the heart.Springer, Berlin Heidelberg New York, p 61–74

Odedra R, Weiss JB (1991) Low molecular weight angiogenesis factor. Pharmacol Ther 49:111–124

Oltman CL, Parker JL, Laughlin MH (1995) Endothelium dependent vasodilation of proximal coronary arteries from exercise-trained pigs. J Appl Physiol 79:33–40

Pearce SC, Hudlická O (1995) Possible involvement of prostaglandins in capillary growth in chronically stimulated skeletal muscles. Microcirculation 2:98

Pipili-Synetos E, Papageorgiou A, Sakkoula E, Sotiropoulou G, Fotsis T, Karakiulakis G, Maragoudakis ME (1995) Inhibition of angiogenesis, tumor-growth and metastasis by the NO-releasing vasodilators, isosorbide mononitrate and dinitrate. Br J Pharmacol 116:1829–1834

Poupa O, Rakusan K, Ostadal B (1970) The effect of physical activity upon the heart of the vertebrates. Med Sport 4:202–235

Price RJ, Skalak TC (1994) Circumferential wall stress as a mechanism for arteriolar rarefaction and proliferation in a network model. Microvasc Res 47:188–202

Price RJ, Owens GK, Skalak TC (1994) Immunohistochemical identification of arteriolar development using markers of smooth muscle differentiation – evidence that capillary arterialization proceeds from terminal arterioles. Circ Res 75:520–527

Przyklenk K, Groom AC (1984) Can exercise promote neovascularisation in the transition zone of infarcted rat hearts? Can J Physiol Pharmacol 62:630–644

Przyklenk K, Groom AC (1985) Effect of exercise frequency, intensity and duration on neovascularization in the transition zone of infarcted rat hearts. Can J Physiol Pharmacol 63:273–278

Rakusan K, Wicker P (1990) Morphometry of the small arteries and arterioles in the rat heart: effects of chronic hypertension and exercise. Cardiovasc Res 24:278–284

Rakusan K, Ostadal B, Wachtlová M (1971) The influence of muscular work on the capillary density in the heart and skeletal muscle of pigeon (Columbia livia dom). Can J Physiol Pharmacol 49:167–170

Regensteiner JG (1997) Exercise in the treatment of claudication: assessment and treatment of functional impairment. Vasc Med 2:238–242

Richardson RS, Mudaliar SRD, Mathieu-Costello O, Wagner PD (1998) VEGF mRNA response to acute exercise following chronic training. Med Sci Sports Exerc 30:S50

Roberts KC, Nixon C, Unthank JL, Lash JM (1997) Femoral artery ligation stimulates capillary growth and limits training-induced increases in oxidative capacity in rats. Microcirculation 4:253–260

Saltin B, Gollnick PD (1983) Skeletal muscle adaptability: significance for metabolism and performance. In: Handbook of physiology, section 10: skeletal muscle. American Physiological Society, Bethesda, p 555–631

Sanne H, Sivertsson R (1968) The effect of exercise on the development of collateral circulation after experimental occlusion of femoral artery in the cat. Acta Physiol Scand 73:257–263

Sasayama S, Fujita M (1992) Recent insights into coronary collateral circulation. Circulation 85:1197–1204

Schamhardt HC, Verdouw PD, Saxena PR (1981) Improvement of perfusion and function of ischemic porcine myocardium after reduction of heart rate by alinidine. J Cardiovasc Pharmacol 3:728–738

Schantz P, Henriksson J, Jansson E (1983) Adaptation of human skeletal muscle to endurance training of long duration. Clin Physiol 3:141–151

Schaper W (1971) The collateral circulation of the heart. North-Holland, Amsterdam

Schaper W, Nienaber C, Gottwick M (1981) The importance of collateral circulation for myocardial survival. Acta Med Scand [Suppl] 657:29–34

Sewell WH, Roth DR (1958) Basic observations on ability of newly formed capillaries to develop into collateral arteries. Surg Forum 9:227–229

Sexton WL, Laughlin MH (1994) Influence of endurance exercise training on distribution of vascular adaptations in rat skeletal muscle. Am J Physiol 266:H483–490

Sexton WL, Korthuis RJ, Laughlin MH (1988) High intensity exercise training increases vascular transport capacity of rat hindquarters. Am J Physiol 254:H274–278

Shammas NW, Moss AJ, Sullebarger JT, Gutierrez OH, Rocco TA (1993) Acquired coronary angiogenesis after myocardial infarction. Cardiology 83:212–216

Sinoway LI, Shenberger J, Wilson J, McLaughlin D, Musch T, Zelis R (1987) A 30-day forearm work protocol increases maximal forearm blood flow. J Appl Physiol 62:1063–1067

Skalak TC, Price RJ (1996) Mechanical stresses in microvascular remodelling. Microcirculation 3:143–165

Skorjanc D, Jaschinski FJ, Heine G, Pette D (1998) Sequential increases in capillarization and mitochondrial enzymes in low-frequency stimulated rabbit muscles. Am J Physiol 274:C810–818

Snell PG, Martin WH, Buckley JC, Blomqvist CG (1987) Maximal vascular leg conductance in trained and untrained men. J Appl Physiol 62:606–610

Spinale FG, Grine RC, Tempel GE, Crawford FA, Zile MR (1992) Alterations in the myocardial capillary vasculature accompany tachycardia induced cardiomyopathy. Basic Res Cardiol 87:65–79

Sun D, Huang A, Koller A, Kaley G (1994) Short term daily exercise activity enhances endothelial NO synthesis in skeletal muscle arterioles of rats. J Appl Physiol 76:2241–2247

Tepperman J, Pearlman D (1961) Effects of exercise and anaemia on coronary arteries of small animals as revealed by the corrosion-cast technique. Circ Res 9:576–584

Tharp GD, Wagner CT (1982) Chronic exercise and cardiac vascularization. Eur J Appl Physiol 48:97–104

Thomas DP (1985) Effects of acute and chronic exercise on myocardial ultrastructure. Med Sci Sports Exerc 17:546–553

Tillmanns H, Ikeda S, Hansen H, Sarma JS, Fauvel JH, Bing RJ (1974) Microcirculation in the ventricle of the dog and turtle. Circ Res 34:561–569

Tillmanns H, Steinhausen M, Leinberger H, Thederan H, Kübler W (1981) Pressure measurement in the terminal vascular bed of the epimyocardium of rats and cats. Circ Res 49:1201–1211

Tillmanns H, Steinhausen M, Leinberger H, Thederan H, Kübler W (1982) The effect of coronary vasodilators on the microcirculation of the ventricular myocardium. In: Tillmanns H, Kübler W, Zebe H (eds) Microcirculation of the heart. Springer, Berlin Heidelberg New York, p 305–312

Tomanek RJ (1970) Effect of age and exercise on the extent of the myocardial capillary bed. Anat Rec 167:55–62

Tomanek RJ (1994) Exercise induced coronary angiogenesis. Med Sci Sports Exerc 26:1245–1251

Tomoike H (1993) Functional aspects of collateral development in animal models. In: Schaper W, Schaper J (eds) Collateral circulation. Kluwer Academic, Boston, p 149–172

Tornling G, Unge G, Skoog L, Ljungqvist A, Carlsson S, Adolfsson J (1978) Proliferative activity of myocardial capillary wall cells in dipyridamole treated rats. Cardiovasc Res 12:692–695

Tsang GMK, Green MA, Crow A, Smith FCT, Beck S, Hudlická O, Shearman CP (1994) Chronic muscle stimulation improves ischemic muscle performance in patients with peripheral vascular disease. Eur J Vasc Surg 8:419–422

Unge G, Carlsson S, Ljungqvist A, Tornling G, Adolfsson J (1979) The proliferative activity of myocardial capillary wall cells in variously aged swimming-exercised rats. Acta Pathol Microbiol Scand [A] Pathol 87:15–17

Valdivia E, Watson M (1960).Histologic alterations in muscles of guinea pigs during chronic hypoxia. Arch Pathol 69:199–208

Wachtlová M, Rakusan K, Poupa O (1965) The coronary terminal vascular bed in the heart of the hare (Lepus Europaeus) and the rabbit (Oryctolagus Domesticus). Physiol Bohemoslov14:328–331

Wachtlová M, Rakusan K, Roth Z, Poupa O (1967) The terminal vascular bed of the myocardium in the wild rat (Rattus Norvegicus) and the laboratory rat (Rattus Norvegicus lab). Physiol Bohemoslov 16:548–554

Ware JA, Simons M (1997) Angiogenesis in ischemic heart disease. Nature Med 3:158–164

White FC, Bloor CM (1995) Coronary growth, not angiogenesis, is the dominant response increasing coronary vascular bed cross-sectional area induced by exercise training. FASEB J 9:A909

White FC, McKirnan M, Breisch EA, Guth BD, Liu Y-M, Bloor CM (1987) Adaptation of the left ventricle to exercise induced hypertrophy. J Appl Physiol 62:1097–1110

White FC, Roth DM, Bloor CM (1990) Coronary vascular remodelling during chronic ischemia. Circulation 82 [Suppl IV]:378

White FC, Bloor CM, McKirnan MD, Caroll SM (1998) Exercise training in swine promotes growth of arteriolar bed and capillary angiogenesis in heart. J Appl Physiol 85:1160–1168

Woodman CR, Muller JM, Laughlin MH, Price EM (1997) Induction of nitric oxide synthase mRNA in coronary resistance arteries isolated from exercise trained rats. Am J Physiol 273:H2575–2579

Wright AJA, Hudlická O (1981) Capillary growth and changes in heart performance induced by chronic bradycardial pacing in the rabbit. Circ Res 49:469–478

Wyatt HL, Mitchell J (1978) Influence of physical conditioning and deconditioning on coronary vasculature of dogs. J Appl Physiol 215:619–625

Xie Z, Gao M, Batra S, Koyama T (1997) The capillarity of left ventricular tissue of rats subjected to coronary artery occlusion. Cardiovasc Res 33:671–676

Yang HT, Ogilvie RW, Terjung RL (1991) Low intensity training produces muscle adaptation in rats with femoral artery stenosis. J Appl Physiol 71:1822–1829

Zetterquist S (1970) Effect of active training on the nutritive blood flow in exercising ischemic legs. Scand J Clin Lab Invest 25:101–111

Zheng W,Tomanek RJ (1998) VEGF is upregulated in bradycardia-induced coronary angiogenesis in rat. FASEB J 12:A71

Zhou A-L, Egginton S (1998) Immunogold labelling of proliferating cells during skeletal muscle angiogenesis. J Vasc Res 35:386

Ziada AMAR, Hudlická O, Tyler KR, Wright AJA (1984) The effect of long-term vasodilation on capillary growth and performance in rabbit heart and skeletal muscle. Cardiovasc Res 18:724–732

Ziada AMAR, Hudlická O, Tyler KR (1989) The effect of long-term administration of a1-blocker prazosin on capillary density in cardiac and skeletal muscle. Pflugers Arch 415:355–360

Ziche M, Morbidelli L, Masini E, Amerini S, Granger HJ, Maggi CA, Geppetti P, Ledda F (1994) Nitric oxide mediates angiogenesis in vivo and endothelial cell growth and migration in vitro promoted by substance P. J Clin Invest 94:2036–2044

7 Myocardial Ischemia and Growth Factor Therapy

M. Simons

7.1 Neovascularization – General Concepts

Neovascularization in mature tissues is a complex process that can lead to development of new, thin-walled vascular structures (angiogenesis) or large-caliber vessels possessing well-developed tunica media (arteriogenesis). Both of these events are a culmination of a number of processes, including dissolution of the existing extracellular matrix, migration and proliferation of endothelial and smooth muscle cells, formation and maturation of new vascular structure, and, finally, deposition of new extracellular matrix (Folkman 1995; Ware and Simons 1997). Clearly, a process of this complexity will have a large number of regulatory check points. Indeed, numerous genes are capable of both stimulation and inhibition of many of the steps involved in regulation. While neovascularization in the heart is usually observed in association with coronary artery disease, other conditions such as hypertrophy or other conditions associated with increased coronary blood flow can also lead to new vessel development (Tomanek and Torry 1994). Furthermore, the concept of ischemia as the primary stimulus of angiogenesis has been recently challenged on the basis of a number experimental observations. For example, chronic reduction of myocardial ischemia with β-blockers had no effect on the development of collateral circulation in the pig ischemia model (Symons et al. 1992). Many cases of advanced coronary disease as well as numerous animal models demonstrate extensive neovascularization around the sites of epicardial coronary artery occlusion. At the same time, either direct or indirect measures of myocardial perfusion fail to document tissue ischemia at these sites. At the same time, few angiographically visible vessels are observed in the distal coronary tree, the site of greatest tissue ischemia. These observations argue that tissue ischemia per se cannot be the sole stimulus for vessel growth. Other stimuli such as shear stress and the presence of local inflammatory response may be key factors involved in control of vessel growth in these settings. In contrast, proliferation of capillaries in the myocardium subtended by the occluded artery may well be stimulated by the presence of tissue ischemia. These considerations suggest, therefore, that different stimuli may account for epicardial (arteriogenesis) versus small intramyocardial (angiogenesis) neovascularization (Schaper and Ito 1996).

7.2 Regulation of the Angiogenic Response

Over the last 5 years, numerous studies in a variety of animal models have examined the ability of angiogenic growth factors to induce physiologically meaningful neovascularization in the setting of chronic ischemia. We and others have observed that several such growth factors (bFGF, aFGF, VEGF), administered either intracoronarily or locally at the site of arterial occlusion , can accelerate new vessel growth in distal parts of the myocardium as well as at sites of epicardial arterial occlusion (Harada et al. 1994, 1996; Lazarous et al. 1995; Lopez et al. 1997b, 1998a,b; Unger et al. 1994). The ability of so many different agents to induce such a complex process successfully suggests either that there are multiple ways of inducing the angiogenic cascade or that, ultimately, the effects of various growth factors converge on a single, common pathway. The necessity to control tightly such a powerful process strongly argues for the latter possibility.

Furthermore, while the effectiveness of such therapy appears to be dose-dependent, at least in the case of bFGF (Lopez et al. 1997), relatively small amounts of these factors reach the myocardium and are retained by it for only a short period of time. However, the observed angiogenic response is very extensive and spans several weeks. These considerations suggest that either these cytokines are unusually potent or their effect on stimulation of angiogenesis has to do with more than just stimulating endothelial cell proliferation. In fact, it is quite likely that the primary effect of such therapy is to set off a cascade of events leading to sustained development of extensive neovascularization. One likely candidate for such a cascade is the stimulation of "inflammatory" response.

Recent discoveries point to association of cardiac and peripheral limb angiogenesis with the presence of "inflammatory" cells and mediators. Thus, expression of monocyte chemoattractant protein-1 (MCP-1) is induced in the endothelium of small venules immediately following reperfusion (Birdsall et al. 1997; Kumar et al. 1997). A local infusion of MCP-1 into an ischemic hind limb also resulted in enhanced collateral growth (Ito et al. 1997). Furthermore, the presence of blood-derived monocytes early after an acute MI was associated with enhanced expression of heparan-sulfate-carrying core proteins (Li et al. 1997) that are involved in regulation of endothelial cell growth. In contrast, the absence of blood-derived monocytes is associated with decreased neovascularization. The ability of macrophages to induce angiogenesis is hardly surprising given the wide variety of cytokines these cells are able to secrete, including VEGF, FGFs, TNFα, Il-6, and Il-8, among others. Studies in a rat acute infarct model suggest that infiltrating macrophages and not myocytes or endothelial cells are the predominant source of VEGF (Li et al. 1996) and, unlike other tissues (Gordon et al. 1995), essentially all cardiac macrophages are of blood-derived (monocyte) origin (Li et al. 1997; Witmer-Pack et al. 1993). VEGF acts as a chemoattractant for macrophages (Barleon et al. 1996) and increases their adhesion to endothelial cells and the extracellular matrix proteins. Thus, a local administration (or production) of VEGF may lead to increased monocyte-macrophage influx followed by release of a number of cytokines including VEGF and bFGF, thus amplifying the original signal. In addition to the cytokine release, macrophages may also be an important source of NO generation that, in turn, can modulate growth factor signaling. In that regard, release of monocyte-derived TNF-α and interleukins will further contribute to generation of NO by stimulating eNOS in endothelial cells. These mechanisms, therefore, may lie at the heart of VEGF-mediated induction of angiogenesis.

In turn, VEGF itself may lie at the center of angiogenic response induced by other cytokines. For example, recent studies in endothelial cell culture and a mouse cornea model of angiogenesis demonstrated FGF-2-dependent induction of VEGF expression in endothelial cells. Furthermore, FGF-2-induced angiogenesis in this study was blocked by anti-VEGF antibodies (Seghezzi et al. 1998). Disruption of the gene for VEGF-A was found to be embryonic-lethal in a heterozygous state (Carmeliet et al. 1996; Ferrara et al. 1996), even though deletions of both alleles of FGF-2 and FGF-5, and double FGF-2/FGF-5 deletions failed to have a significant effect on angiogenesis (Zhou et al. 1998). In addition to VEGF, PDGF may represent another key mediator of angiogenesis, perhaps particularly in the myocardium (Edelberg et al. 1998). Deletion of the gene for PDGFRα leads to mutants showing vascular ruptures and diminished numbers of smooth muscle cells (Schatteman et al. 1992), while the PDGFRβ knockout mice show abnormalities in capillary organization and shape (Soriano 1994).

Other key proteins in vascular development and perhaps in neovascularization in adult tissues include tissue factor (TF), thrombomodulin (TM), TIE-1, TIE-2 and its ligands, angiopoietins 1 and 2, and TGF-β. Knockout mice studies in the case of each of these genes have demonstrated profound alterations in vascular development.

In addition to growth factors, a number of other molecules, including Il-6, IL-8, PAF, substance P, nitric oxide (NO), and adenosine have been implicated to have the ability to stimulate angiogenesis. In particular, administration of adenosine has been associated with evidence of angiogenic response in animal models (Granger et al. 1994; Hashimoto et al. 1994; Takagi et al. 1996). The mechanism of action of these molecules remains poorly understood at present. NO has the ability to stimulate or suppress proliferation and migration of a variety of cell types, including smooth muscle and endothelial cells, as well as to activate expression of various inflammatory cytokines. There appears to be a connection between NO production and blood vessel growth. For example VEGF, FGF, and substance-P all stimulate NO release and are associated with development of neovascularization in vivo (Montrucchio et al. 1997; Murohara et al. 1998; Parenti et al. 1998; Ziche et al. 1994, 1997). Proliferative effects of VEGF in cell culture and the ability of TGF-β to induce vessel formation in 3D gels is suppressed by NO synthase inhibitors. Thus, NO generation may be a key event in angiogenesis. In this regard, it is particularly interesting to note defective angiogenesis in a peripheral limb ischemia model in the eNOS knockout mouse (Murohara et al. 1998).

7.3 Animal Studies of Coronary Angiogenesis

To date, a number of growth factors, including FGF-1, FGF-2, FGF-4, FGF-5, VEGF-A, and HGF have been shown to possess the ability to induce new vessel growth in mature adult tissues. The ability of FGF-2 to induce significant angiogenesis in mature tissues was suggested by studies in canine and porcine infarction models that demonstrated increased peri-infarct vessel formation in a setting of FGF-2 administration (Battler et al. 1993; Yanagisawa-Miwa et al. 1992). Initial studies of the therapeutic efficacy of FGF-2 in chronic myocardial ischemia suggested that prolonged administration either of daily injections (110 μg of FGF-2 for 18 days) into the circumflex coronary artery distally to an ameroid occluder, or of daily left atrial injections (1.74 mg of FGF-2 for 18 days), result in early augmentation of coronary flow to the compromised territory and were associated with histological evidence of angiogenesis (Lazarous et al. 1995; Unger et al. 1994). However, continued FGF-2 administration beyond 18 days (for up to 6 months) did not result in a further increase in collateral blood flow, which also applied to FGF-2- and saline-treated animals (Lazarous et al. 1995). Despite promising results, these studies were compromised by the need for very high amounts of FGF-2 and the lack of evaluation of physiological benefit of increased collateral development.

Local perivascular delivery of FGF-2 using heparin-alginate microspheres was evaluated in a porcine model of chronic myocardial ischemia (LCX ameroid occlusion). Heparin-alginate delivery provides zero-order release kinetics of FGF-2 from the polymer over a 4–5 week period, and the implantation of the beads is not associated with any inflammatory reaction (Edelman et al. 1991, 1993; Lopez et al. 1996). Perivascular delivery has the potential advantage of bypassing the endothelial barrier, so avoiding rapid washout of the growth factor due to rapid arterial blood flow. In these studies, delivery of approximately 5 μg of FGF-2 leads to significantly better preservation of perfusion of the ischemic zone during pacing, compared with control animals, as well as to better preservation of the regional left ventricular function (Harada et al. 1994). Examination of the effects of progressively larger amounts of FGF-2 (10 μgand 100 μg respectively) delivered similarly in a pig model (Lopez et al. 1997) demonstrated dose-dependent improvement of coronary perfusion accompanied by an improvement in left ventricular function. In addition to improving angiographic collaterals, myocardial perfusion, and left ventricular function, perivascular delivery of FGF-2 resulted in normalization of ischemia-induced impairment of endothelium-dependent vasodilation in the ischemic area of the left circumflex coronary artery (Sellke et al. 1994, 1995).

All attempts to stimulate myocardial angiogenesis discussed so far have employed prolonged growth factor delivery. However, single-dose delivery is clearly preferable from a patient care standpoint. To this end, several investigators have explored the utility of intrapericardial delivery of FGF-2. Studies in a porcine ameroid model demonstrated that a single intrapericardial injection of FGF-2 results in significant dose-dependent increases in the left-to-left angiographic collateral index and myocardial blood flow in the ameroid-compromised territory blood flow, which was accompanied by improvements in regional myocardial function as well as histologic evidence of increased myocardial vascularity. None of these benefits were seen in saline- or heparin-treated ischemic animals (Laham et al. 1998). Similar results were obtained in two other animal models (Landau et al. 1995; Uchida et al. 1995). Similar animal studies also demonstrated the physiological benefit of FGF-1 and FGF-5 therapy (Giordano et al. 1996; Lopez et al. 1998a; Tabata et al. 1997).

Of the major isoforms of VEGF-A ($VEGF_{121}$, $VEGF_{165}$, $VEGF_{189}$, and $VEGF_{206}$), the majority of studies have concentrated on $VEGF_{165}$, although $VEGF_{121}$ has recently been receiving increasing attention. Despite its obvious importance in angiogenesis, initial studies of therapeutic applications of VEGF-A in the heart produced somewhat ambiguous results.

A study carried out in a dog ameroid model using daily intracoronary injections of 45 μg of VEGF delivered distally to the occluder over a 28 day period (total dose: 900 μg) demonstrated faster restoration of collateral zone flow in the test group compared to the saline control group (Banai et al. 1994). Morphological analysis demonstrated a significantly higher number of small (20 μm diameter) vessels, but no change in the number of capillaries in VEGF-treated animal compared to the control group. However, a subsequent study by the same group of investigators using an identical model failed to show any beneficial effect of a 7 day course of VEGF infusions (total dose 720 μg) (Lazarous et al. 1996). It is not clear why there was such a dramatic difference between the two studies; reduction of the total dose and a shorter duration of infusion in the second study may have played a role.

Perivascular delivery of VEGF was tested in the porcine model using an implantable minipump containing 2 μg of VEGF and 50 U of heparin, positioned periadventitially to the circumflex coronary artery and distal to the ameroid occluder (Harada et al. 1996). Heparin alone was infused into control animals. Comparison of VEGF/heparin- and heparin-treated groups showed that while coronary flow in the ischemic territory at rest was no different between the two groups, VEGF treatment was associated with better coronary flow during pacing. MRI demonstrated significantly better perfusion of the ameroid territory in the VEGF-treated group (Pearlman et al. 1995). Morphometric analysis found a nearly fourfold increase in the number of collateral vessels in VEGF-treated animals that was limited to the ischemic zone (Harada et al. 1996). Myocardial ischemia is predominantly a subendocardial event characterized by a decrease in the subendocardial-to-subepicardial blood flow ratio (Q_{endo}/Q_{epi}). Interestingly, despite periadventitial administration of VEGF in this study, examination of subendocardial and subepicardial flows showed that, while at rest there was no difference in the transmyocardial blood flow distribution (Q_{endo}/Q_{epi}) in the compromised myocardia of VEGF-treated and control animals during pacing, subendocardial flow in the control group fell significantly compared to that of the VEGF group. Thus, epicardial administration of the growth factor resulted in significantly better preservation of transmyocardial flow distribution during pacing stress (Harada et al. 1996).

As in FGF-1 and FGF-2 studies, improvements in coronary perfusion associated with VEGF therapy were accompanied by significantly better restoration of endothelium-mediated, receptor-dependent relaxation in the microcirculation of VEGF-treated animals. These improvements in coronary flow and microvascular function were reflected in enhanced left ventricular performance in VEGF-treated animals, as demonstrated by a higher ejection fraction and better preservation of regional wall shortening during pacing stress (Harada et al. 1996).

The feasibility of single bolus intracoronary VEGF delivery was tested by Hariawala et al. (1996), who injected 2 mg of $rhVEGF_{165}$ into the left coronary artery of eight pigs. Four of the eight animals survived the injection (with four dying of acute refractory hypotension); however, 30 days later, the remaining animals demonstrated improved coronary flow as compared to the control group (Hariawala et al. 1996). Given a 50% mortality of high-dose single bolus VEGF therapy, a lower dose (20 μg) single bolus intracoronary injection was compared in efficacy to the same amount of VEGF delivered either perivascularly or locally using an InfusaSleeve (LocalMed, Palo Alto, Calif.). The studies conducted in a porcine model demonstrated that both intracoronary bolus injection and local delivery resulted in significant increase of angiographically visible left-to-left, but not right-to-left, collaterals, and improvement in myocardial blood flow and regional left ventricular function. Although there was a trend towards better results with local delivery as compared to intracoronary bolus delivery, both methods appeared equally efficacious. There was no significant hemodynamic compromise associated with any of these delivery approaches (Lopez et al. 1998).

Thus, VEGF, delivered by either intracoronary or periadventitial methods appears to be an effective angiogenic agent. As suggested by coronary angiography, the cytokine seems to induce both tissue angiogenesis (as documented by increased vessel counts) as well as neoarteriogenesis at the occlusion site.

7.4 Coronary Microcirculation and Hemodynamics

While most animal studies of coronary angiogenesis have focused on evaluation of coronary flow and function, another key aspect of growth factor activity is their effects on microcirculation. Microvessels from the chronically ischemic pig myocardium demonstrate reduced vasodilation to endothelium receptor-dependent agonists such as ADP and serotonin, but not to non-endothelium-dependent agents such as A23187. Vasodilation was fully restored following administration of VEGF, bFGF, or aFGF (Harada et al. 1996; Sellke et al. 1994, 1996a). At the same time, microvessels from chronically ischemic myocardium demonstrated enhanced ability to vasodilate in response to VEGF and bFGF in comparison to microvessels from nonischemic tissues (Sellke et al. 1996). The latter finding appears to be due to higher levels of expression of iNOS in the ischemic tissues as well as increased expression of VEGF and FGF receptors (Sellke et al. 1996a, b). In the course of these studies, we and others (Hariawala et al. 1996) noted significant systemic hypotension induced by VEGF administration. To define this effect better and to explore its mechanism, we carried out a detailed hemodynamic evaluation of intracoronary VEGF administration in pigs. We found that VEGF produced a dose-dependent increase in coronary blood flow followed by a steep decline in systemic vascular resistance. In fact, VEGF was as potent a coronary vasodilator as maximal doses of adenosine, without displaying any of the negative chronotropic effects associated with the latter. The ability of VEGF to increase coronary flow was largely but not fully blocked by inhibitors of NO synthase. An unexpected finding was the induction of tachyphylaxis to coronary vasodilator effects of VEGF during repeat growth factor administrations (Lopez et al. 1997). Observations using intravascular ultrasound during intracoronary VEGF infusion suggested that most of this cytokine's vasodilating effects involve small vessels rather than large epicardial arteries. This finding has been confirmed in ex vivo studies of coronary rings and microvessels, and appears to be largely due to enhanced VEGF ability to generate NO in microvasculature (30–100 μm) compared to larger arterioles (Laham et al. 1997).

7.5 Tracking Angiogenesis – The Role of MR Imaging

The ability to assess changes in myocardial perfusion over time is a key to successful evaluation of angiogenic agents in clinical trials. However, nuclear perfusion imaging, the usual means of perfusion studies, suffers from a number of limitations that probably render it insufficient for these studies. In particular, nuclear perfusion imaging relies on relative assessment of normal and abnormal areas. A change in perfusion of the "normal" territory can make results of even quantitative assessment grossly inaccurate. This concern is heightened in patients with multivessel coronary disease – typically forming the majority in early angiogenic trials. While it is debatable whether normal perfusion areas actually exist in this patient population, it is easy to imagine that a growth factor may induce changes in perfusion in both "normal" as well as "target" areas. While the ability of growth factors to induce angiogenesis is clearly lower in normal tissues, it still is not entirely lacking (Giordano et al. 1996; Muhlhauser et al. 1995a,b; Pili et al. 1997). The other limitation of nuclear perfusion imaging is its relatively poor spatial resolution, which renders it insensitive to small and moderate changes in perfusion.

An imaging modality that has recently shown considerable promise in noninvasive assessment of coronary blood flow is magnetic resonance (MR) perfusion imaging. MR perfusion imaging relies on assessment of a T1-sensitive contrast signal in the myocardium. In this form of MR imaging, the contrast density is not indexed to the "normal" part of the myocardium, but to the left ventricular cavity. The technique then estimates both a degree of delay of the contrast arrival to the ischemic zone and an area (or volume) of the myocardium demonstrating delayed flow arrival (Pearlman et al. 1995). The major technical limitation of this approach is the need for a relatively tight contrast bolus that can achieved by forceful intravenous injection. Application of this approach in animal studies demonstrating delayed contrast arrival in the ameroid-compromised zone and its size as determined by MR correlated closely with morphological measurements (Pearlman et al. 1995). Studies in the pig model demonstrated that this method could accurately identify and quantify the therapeutic benefit of VEGF administration (Pearlman et al. 1995).

A second MR-based technique recently developed by our group allows tracking of the developing collateral circulation. This approach relies on detection of heterogeneous distribution of the T2 signal in local magnetic field gradients. The signal generated by the susceptibility contrast agent arrival at a tissue supplied by sparsely distributed small vessels is different from the signal generated by a contrast agent arriving via a normal vessel network, and can be detected in T2-weighted images as a transient drop in signal intensity. Our preliminary studies using T2-weighted images with added preparation pulses used to emphasize T2 contrast have demonstrated that it is indeed possible to detect a signal difference between tissues supplied by normal and collateral vessel networks (JD Pearlman, RJ Laham, M. Simons, unpublished observations). This approach to MR image generation produced a clearly visible "dark flash" area corresponding to the location of collateral-supplied tissues in the heart.

To demonstrate the accuracy of this approach, we compared the MR-determined extent of collateral territory to the ex vivo images generated by 3D elastic subtraction CT imaging (Pearlman et al. 1997) obtained after direct intracoronary contrast injection. There was a remarkable visual similarity between both sets of images; and quantitative analysis of the territory extent also demonstrated close correlation between the two techniques (r^2=0.98). Similarly, comparing the MR-determined extent of collateral perfusion to coronary microsphere data also demonstrated a close correlation between the techniques (r^2=0.86). Thus, newly developed collateral-sensitive MR imaging (CS-MR) provides accurate assessment of the collateral perfusion zone in live animals.

7.6 Clinical Studies of Coronary Angiogenesis

Given observations in a variety of animal studies, the stage has been set for clinical studies of coronary angiogenesis (Table 1). In studies published to date, injection of FGF-1 at the site of LIMA to LAD anastomosis has been found to be safe and to potentially promote formation of a local collateral network (Schumacher et al. 1998). In another study, insertion of FGF-2 in heparin-alginate pellets into areas of the myocardium not revascularized at the time of CABG was found to be techni-

Table 1. Clinical studies of coronary angiogenesis

Growth Factor	Delivery	Type	Phase	Sponsor	Status
FGF-1	Intramyocardial	Protein	I	——	Completed
FGF-2	Intracoronary	Protein	I	Chiron	Completed
FGF-2	Perivascular	Protein	I	NIH	Completed
FGF-2	Intravenous	Protein	I	Chiron	Completed
FGF-2	Intracoronary	Protein	II	Chiron	Ongoing
FGF-2	Perivascular	Protein	II	NIH	Ongoing
FGF-4	Intracoronary	Adenovirus	I	Collat Ther/ Berlex	Ongoing
VEGF-A165	Intracoronary	Protein	I	Genentech	Completed
VEGF-A165	Intravenous	Protein	I	Genentech	Completed
VEGF-A165	Intracoronary/ intravenous	Protein	II	Genentech	Completed
VEGF-A165	Intracoronary	Adenovirus	I	——	Completed
VEGF-A165	Intramyocardial	Plasmid	I	Isner	Ongoing
VEGF-A121	Intramyocardial	Adenovirus	I	GenVec	Ongoing

cally feasible and safe (Sellke et al. 1998). In particular, there were no detectable systemic levels of FGF-2 nor any hemodynamic compromise associated with growth factor delivery. Preliminary results suggest improvement in myocardial perfusion in patients treated with FGF-2 as compared to placebo-treated controls (Sellke et al. 1998). Other ongoing surgical studies are evaluating intramyocardial injections of adenoviral vectors or naked DNA encoding $VEGF_{121}$ and VEGF-A. In addition, a number of catheter-based studies are evaluating the efficacy of intracoronary or intravenous administration of VEGF-A, FGF-2, and FGF-4 in protein-based or gene-therapy-based approaches. Phase I studies of intracoronary $VEGF_{165}$ and FGF-2 administration have already been completed and phase II studies are in progress. Already on the horizon are the next generation of agents that promise to be more powerful than the growth factors currently being tested.

The choice of end points in these studies will become critical for assessment of efficacy and demonstration of mechanisms of growth factor benefits. Early results suggest improvement in symptoms and exercise time. However, to date there has been no convincing demonstration of functional improvement or improvements in myocardial perfusion as assessed by nuclear imaging. In fact, these studies appear to parallel closely the experience with laser myocardial revascularization trials that have also demonstrated improvements in symptoms and exercise time that are not displayed on nuclear myocardial perfusion imaging. Since virtually all of the early growth factor studies are unblinded and the patients recruited tend to be highly motivated, it is difficult to assess the significance of the observed improvements in such "soft" end points as symptoms and exercise duration. Consequently, it will be critical for subsequent studies to assess such "hard" end points as LV function, myocardial perfusion, and survival (or freedom from revascularization). As already discussed, it is uncertain whether nuclear imaging will be sufficient for documenting changes in myocardial perfusion. In addition to nuclear perfusion imaging, MR or positron emission tomography (PET), assessment of angiogenesis may also prove useful in these studies because of their ability to identify and quantify the extent of underperfused myocardium. Coronary angiography may provide information regarding the development of angiographically visible collaterals as well as potential progression of underlying coronary disease.

7.7 Choice of Growth Factor and Method of Delivery

Given a variety of different approaches to stimulation of coronary angiogenesis that have been tested in preclinical studies, a number of important questions arise regarding the choice of growth factor, mode of delivery, and relative benefit of gene transfer versus protein infusion. While a number of growth factors have been shown to date that are capable of inducing physiologically significant angiogenesis, no study has carried out a direct head-to head comparison of these cytokines. Furthermore, several cell culture level studies suggest synergistic relationships between some of these factors (Asahara et al. 1995; Pepper et al. 1992). In the final analysis, if all of these factors appear relatively equipotent, the final choice of growth factor may well be determined by issues such as ease of use and the frequency and severity of side effects.

While the use of an endothelial-specific growth factor such as VEGF has theoretical advantages over growth factors with more widespread targets, such as FGF, given the documented ability of these factors to induce expression of each other, such considerations are likely to be more theoretical than practical because of the wish to avoid undesired mitogenesis.

The choice of delivery strategy is ultimately dictated by efficacy, safety, and patient convenience considerations. With regard to the latter, single bolus intravenous administration would clearly be the most advantageous. However, to date there are only limited data regarding the efficacy of this mode of delivery. Single bolus intracoronary administration appears effective for both FGF-2 and $VEGF_{165}$, although with VEGF the dose is limited by systemic hypotension. In one animal study, intracoronary injection appeared fairly similar to local intracoronary or sustained release perivascular delivery (Lopez et al. 1998).

As it seems most prudent to induce angiogenesis only in the region of myocardial ischemia, and to use as low a concentration of angiogenic growth factors as is feasible, the fact that significant physiological effects have been achieved with extracoronary delivery using much smaller amounts of growth factors than those used for intracoronary or intra-arterial approaches is potentially exciting. This consideration is balanced, however, by the need for a surgical manipulation to achieve such delivery. Thus, perivascular delivery may find its best application in surgical cases, if an angiogenic growth factor is used in conjunction with bypass surgery.

7.8 Future and Prognosis

In addition to the problems related to nonspecific mitogenesis, several other potential limitations for angiogenesis-based therapy have been considered, including potentiation of angiogenesis-driven diseases such as diabetic retinopathy and certain tumors. In particular, diabetic retinopathy is associated with the presence of VEGF in the vitreous humor (Aiello et al. 1994), and administration of VEGF-neutralizing antibodies arrests the process in experimental animals. By virtue of its effect on vessel permeability, VEGF might also lead to exacerbation or initiation of local edema and inflammatory reactions. Furthermore, because of the cytokine's prominent vasoactive properties, substantial systemic hypotension may present dose-limiting toxicity. It is of note that, in limited clinical experience, plasmid-mediated VEGF gene therapy led to development of extensive extremity edema and telangiectasia in a patient to whom the expression construct was administered intra-arterially in the leg (Isner et al. 1996). Administration of basic FGF in high dosages is also associated with a number of side effects, including anemia, thrombocytopenia, membranous nephropathy, and hyperostosis (Mazue et al. 1991).

One more theoretical concern is that VEGF and FGFs may exacerbate plaque angiogenesis and thus adversely affect plaque stability or progression of atherosclerotic coronary disease. In particular, VEGF's promotion of permeability could theoretically lead to plaque expansion or rupture, since intraplaque vessels tend to be quite permeable, even without exogenous VEGF. In addition, these growth factors might stimulate progression of coronary stenosis by stimulating growth of fibroblasts and medial smooth muscle cells. For instance, prolonged infusion of VEGF has been associated with increased progression of post-angioplasty restenosis in a recent study in dogs (Lazarous et al. 1996), although other studies have not demonstrated this effect.

Clearly, this is a new and unexplored territory. Just as clearly, therapeutic angiogenesis, alone or in combination with laser-based revascularization, promises a paradigm change in approach to patients with ischemic heart disease. While there is tremendous hope, there must also be considerable caution, since our understanding of the biology of angiogenesis and the mechanism of growth factor activity still leave much to be desired. The results of clinical studies over the next few years will determine the place and role of this kind of therapy.

References

Aiello LP, Avery RL, Arrigg PG, Keyt BA, Jampel HD, Shah ST, Pasquale LR, Thieme H, Iwamoto MA, Park JE (1994) Vascular endothelial growth factor in ocular fluid of patients with diabetic retinopathy and other retinal disorders (see comments). N Engl J Med 331:1480–1487

Asahara T, Bauters C, Zheng LP, Takeshita S, Bunting S, Ferrara N, Symes JF, Isner JM (1995) Synergistic effect of vascular endothelial growth factor and basic fibroblast growth factor on angiogenesis in vivo. Circulation 92:II365–371

Banai S, Jaklitsch MT, Shou M, Lazarous DF, Scheinowitz M, Biro S, Epstein SE, Unger EF (1994) Angiogenic-induced enhancement of collateral blood flow to ischemic myocardium by vascular endothelial growth factor in dogs. Circulation 89:2183–2189

Barleon B, Sozzani S, Zhou D, Weich HA, Mantovani A, Marme D(1996) Migration of human monocytes in response to vascular endothelial growth factor (VEGF) is mediated via the VEGF receptor flt-1. Blood 87:3336–3343

Battler A, Scheinowitz M, Bor A, Hasdai D, Vered Z, Di Segni E, Varda-Bloom N, Nass D, Engelberg S, Eldar M et al. (1993) Intracoronary injection of basic fibroblast growth factor enhances angiogenesis in infarcted swine myocardium. J Am Coll Cardiol 22:2001–2006

Birdsall HH, Green DM, Trial J, Youker KA, Burns AR, MacKay CR, LaRosa GJ, Hawkins HK, Smith CW, Michael LH, Entman ML, Rossen RD (1997) Complement C5a, TGF-beta 1, and MCP-1, in sequence, induce migration of monocytes into ischemic canine myocardium within the first one to five hours after reperfusion. Circulation 95:684–692

Carmeliet P, Ferreira V, Breier G, Pollefeyt S, Kieckens L, Gertsenstein M, Fahrig M, Vandenhoeck A, Harpal K, Eberhardt C, Declercq C, Pawling J, Moons L, Collen D, Risau W, Nagy A (1996) Abnormal blood vessel development and lethality in embryos lacking a single VEGF allele. Nature 380:435–439

Edelberg JM, Aird WC, Wu W, Rayburn H, Mamuya WS, Mercola M, Rosenberg RD (1998) PDGF mediates cardiac microvascular communication (in process citation). J Clin Invest 102:837–843

Edelman ER, Mathiowitz E, Langer R, Klagsbrun M (1991) Controlled and modulated release of basic fibroblast growth factor. Biomaterials 12:619–626

Edelman ER, Nugent MA, Karnovsky MJ (1993) Perivascular and intravenous administration of basic fibroblast growth factor: vascular and solid organ deposition. Proc Natl Acad Sci USA 90:1513–1517

Ferrara N, Carver-Moore K, Chen H, Dowd M, Lu L, KS OS, Powell-Braxton L, Hillan KJ, Moore MW (1996) Heterozygous embryonic lethality induced by targeted inactivation of the VEGF gene. Nature 380:439–442

Folkman J (1995) Angiogenesis in cancer, vascular, rheumatoid and other disease. Nat Med 1:27–31

Giordano FJ, Ping P, McKirnan MD, Nozaki S, DeMaria AN, Dillmann WH, Mathieu-Costello O, Hammond HK (1996) Intracoronary transfer of fibroblast growth factor-5 increases blood flow and contractile function in an ischemic region of the heart. Nat Med 2:534–539

Gordon S, Clarke S, Greaves D, Doyle A (1995) Molecular immunobiology of macrophages: recent progress. Curr Opin Immunol 7:24–33

Granger HJ, Ziche M, Hawker JR Jr, Meininger CJ, Czisny LE, Zawieja DC (1994) Molecular and cellular basis of myocardial angiogenesis. Cell Mol Biol Res 40:81–85

Harada K, Grossman W, Friedman M, Edelman ER, Prasad PV, Keighley CS, Manning WJ, Sellke FW, Simons M (1994) Basic fibroblast growth factor improves myocardial function in chronically ischemic porcine hearts. J Clin Invest 94:623–630

Harada K, Friedman M, Lopez JJ, Wang SY, Li J, Prasad PV, Pearlman JD, Edelman ER, Sellke FW, Simons M (1996) Vascular endothelial growth factor administration in chronic myocardial ischemia. Am J Physiol 270:H1791–802

Hariawala MD, Horowitz JJ, Esakof D, Sheriff DD, Walter DH, Keyt B, Isner JM, Symes JF (1996) VEGF improves myocardial blood flow but produces EDRF-mediated hypotension in porcine hearts. J Surg Res 63:77–82

Hashimoto E, Kage K, Ogita T, Nakaoka T, Matsuoka R, Kira Y (1994) Adenosine as an endogenous mediator of hypoxia for induction of vascular endothelial growth factor mRNA in U-937 cells. Biochem Biophys Res Commun 204:318–324

Isner JM, Pieczek A, Schainfeld R, Blair R, Haley L, Asahara T, Rosenfield K, Razvi S, Walsh K, Symes JF (1996) Clinical evidence of angiogenesis after arterial gene transfer of phVEGF165 in patient with ischaemic limb. Lancet 348:370–374

Ito WD, Arras M, Winkler B, Scholz D, Schaper J, Schaper W (1997) Monocyte chemotactic protein-1 increases collateral and peripheral conductance after femoral artery occlusion. Circ Res 80:829–837

Kumar AG, Ballantyne CM, Michael LH, Kukielka GL, Youker KA, Lindsey ML, Hawkins HK, Birdsall HH, MacKay CR, LaRosa GJ, Rossen RD, Smith CW, Entman ML (1997) Induction of monocyte chemoattractant protein-1 in the small veins of the ischemic and reperfused canine myocardium. Circulation 95:693–700

Laham R, Tofukuji M, Sellke F, Simons M (1997) Vascular endothelial growth factor (VEGF) affects microvessels bu not epicardial arteries and veins. Circulation 96:I-551

Laham R, Sellke F, Edelman J, Simons M (1998) Local perivascular basic fibroblast growth factor (bFGF) treatment in patients with ischemic heart disease. J Am Coll Cardiol 31:394A

Landau C, Jacobs AK, Haudenschild CC (1995) Intrapericardial basic fibroblast growth factor induces myocardial angiogenesis in a rabbit model of chronic ischemia. Am Heart J 129:924–931

Lazarous DF, Scheinowitz M, Shou M, Hodge E, Rajanayagam S, Hunsberger S, Robison WG, Jr, Stiber JA, Correa R, Epstein SE et al. (1995) Effects of chronic systemic administration of basic fibroblast growth factor on collateral development in the canine heart. Circulation 91:145–153

Lazarous DF, Shou M, Scheinowitz M, Hodge E, Thirumurti V, Kitsiou AN, Stiber JA, Lobo AD, Hunsberger S, Guetta E, Epstein SE, Unger EF (1996) Comparative effects of basic fibroblast growth factor and vascular endothelial growth factor on coronary collateral development and the arterial response to injury. Circulation 94:1074–1082

Li J, Brown LF, Hibberd MG, Grossman JD, Morgan JP, Simons M (1996) VEGF, flk-1, and flt-1 expression in a rat myocardial infarction model of angiogenesis. Am J Physiol 270:H1803–H1811

Li J, Brown LF, Laham RJ, Volk R, Simons M (1997) Macrophage-dependent regulation of syndecan gene expression. Circ Res 81:785–796

Lopez J, Edelman E, Stamler A, Morgan J, Sellke F, Simons M (1996) Local perivascular administration of basic fibroblast growth factor: drug delivery and toxicological evalaution. Drug Metab Dispos 24:922–924

Lopez J, Laham RJ, Carrozza JC, Tofukuji M, Sellke FW, Bunting S, Simons M (1997a) Hemodynamic effects of intracoronary VEGF delivery: evidence of tachyphylaxis and NO dependence of response. Am J Physiol 273:H1317–1323

Lopez JJ, Edelman ER, Stamler A, Hibberd MG, Prasad P, Caputo RP, Carrozza JC, Douglas PS, Sellke FW, Simons M (1997b) Basic fibroblast growth factor in a porcine model of chronic myocardial ischemia: a comparison of angiographic, echocardiographic and coronary flow parameters. J Pharmacol Exp Ther 282:385–390

Lopez JJ, Edelman ER, Stamler A, Hibberd MG, Prasad P, Thomas KA, DiSalvo J, Caputo RP, Carrozza JP, Douglas PS, Sellke FW, Simons M (1998a) Angiogenic potential of perivascularly delivered aFGF in a porcine model of chronic myocardial ischemia. Am J Physiol 274:H930–936

Lopez JJ, Laham RJ, Stamler A, Pearlman JD, Bunting S, Kaplan A, Carrozza JP, Sellke FW, Simons M (1998b) VEGF administration in chronic myocardial ischemia in pigs. Cardiovasc Res 40:272–281

Mazue G, Bertolero F, Jacob C, Sarmientos P, Roncucci R (1991) Preclinical and clinical studies with recombinant human basic fibroblast growth factor. Ann NY Acad Sci 638:329–340

Montrucchio G, Lupia E, de Martino A, Battaglia E, Arese M, Tizzani A, Bussolino F, Camussi G (1997) Nitric oxide mediates angiogenesis induced in vivo by platelet- activating factor and tumor necrosis factor-alpha. Am J Pathol 151:557–563

Muhlhauser J, Merrill MJ, Pili R, Maeda H, Bacic M, Bewig B, Passaniti A, Edwards NA, Crystal RG, Capogrossi MC (1995a) VEGF165 expressed by a replication-deficient recombinant adenovirus vector induces angiogenesis in vivo. Circ Res 77:1077–1086

Muhlhauser J, Pili R, Merrill MJ, Maeda H, Passaniti A, Crystal RG, Capogrossi MC (1995b) In vivo angiogenesis induced by recombinant adenovirus vectors coding either for secreted or nonsecreted forms of acidic fibroblast growth factor. Hum Gene Ther 6:1457–1465

Murohara T, Asahara T, Silver M, Bauters C, Masuda H, Kalka C, Kearney M, Chen D, Symes JF, Fishman MC, Huang PL, Isner JM (1998) Nitric oxide synthase modulates angiogenesis in response to tissue ischemia. J Clin Invest 101:2567–2578

Parenti A, Morbidelli L, Cui XL, Douglas JG, Hood JD, Granger HJ, Ledda F, Ziche M (1998) Nitric oxide is an upstream signal of vascular endothelial growth factor-induced extracellular signal-regulated kinase1/2 activation in postcapillary endothelium. J Biol Chem 273:4220–4226

Pearlman JD, Hibberd MG, Chuang ML, Harada K, Lopez JJ, Gladstone SR, Friedman M, Sellke FW, Simons M (1995) Magnetic resonance mapping demonstrates benefits of VEGF-induced myocardial angiogenesis. Nat Med 1:1085–1089

Pearlman JD, Laham RJ, Simons M, Gladstone S, Raptopoulos V (1997) Extent of myocardial collateralization: determination with three- dimensional elastic-subtraction spiral CT. Acad Radiol 4:680–686

Pepper MS, Ferrara N, Orci L, Montesano R (1992) Potent synergism between vascular endothelial growth factor and basic fibroblast growth factor in the induction of angiogenesis in vitro. Biochem Biophys Res Commun 189:824–831

Pili R, Chang J, Muhlhauser J, Crystal RG, Capogrossi MC, Passaniti A (1997) Adenovirus-mediated gene transfer of fibroblast growth factor-1: angiogenesis and tumorigenicity in nude mice. Int J Cancer 73:258–263

Schaper W, Ito W (1996) Molecular mechanisms of collateral vessel growth. Circ Res 79:911–919

Schatteman GC, Morrison-Graham K, van Koppen A, Weston JA, Bowen-Pope DF (1992) Regulation and role of PDGF receptor alpha-subunit expression during embryogenesis. Development 115:123–131

Schumacher B, Pecher P, von Specht B, Stegmann T (1998) Induction of neoangiogenesis in ischemic myocardium by human growth factors. Circulation 97:645–650

Seghezzi G, Patel S, Ren CJ, Gualandris A, Pintucci G, Robbins ES, Shapiro RL, Galloway AC, Rifkin DB, Mignatti P (1998) Fibroblast growth factor-2 (FGF-2) induces vascular endothelial growth factor (VEGF) expression in the endothelial cells of forming capillaries: an autocrine mechanism contributing to angiogenesis. J Cell Biol 141:1659–1673

Sellke FW, Wang SY, Friedman M, Harada K, Edelman ER, Grossman W, Simons M (1994) Basic FGF enhances endothelium-dependent relaxation of the collateral- perfused coronary microcirculation. Am J Physiol 267:H1303–1311

Sellke FW, Wang SY, Friedman M, Dai HB, Harada K, Lopez JJ, Simons M (1995) Beta-adrenergic modulation of the collateral-dependent coronary microcirculation. J Surg Res 59:185–190

Sellke FW, Li J, Stamler A, Lopez JJ, Thomas KA, Simons M (1996a) Angiogenesis induced by acidic fibroblast growth factor as an alternative method of revascularization for chronic myocardial ischemia. Surgery 120:182–188

Sellke FW, Wang SY, Stamler A, Lopez JJ, Li J, LI J, Simons M (1996b) Enhanced microvascular relaxations to VEGF and bFGF in chronically ischemic porcine myocardium. Am J Physiol 271:H713–720

Sellke FW, Laham RJ, Edelman ER, Pearlman JD, Simons M (1998) Therapeutic angiogenesis with basic fibroblast growth factor: technique and early results. Ann Thorac Surg 65:1540–1544

Soriano P (1994) Abnormal kidney development and hematological disorders in PDGF beta- receptor mutant mice. Genes Dev 8:1888–1896

Symons JD, Pitsillides KF, Longhurst JC (1992) Chronic reduction of myocardial ischemia does not attenuate coronary collateral development in miniswine. Circulation 86:660–671

Tabata H, Silver M, Isner JM (1997) Arterial gene transfer of acidic fibroblast growth factor for therapeutic angiogenesis in vivo: critical role of secretion signal in use of naked DNA. Cardiovasc Res 35:470–479

Takagi H, King GL, Ferrara N, Aiello LP (1996) Hypoxia regulates vascular endothelial growth factor receptor KDR/Flk gene expression through adenosine A2 receptors in retinal capillary endothelial cells. Invest Ophthalmol Vis Sci 37:1311–1321

Tomanek R, Torry R (1994) Growth of coronary vasculature in hypertrophy; mechanism and model dependence. Cell Mol Biol Res 1994:129–136

Uchida Y, Yanagisawa-Miwa A, Nakamura F, Yamada K, Tomaru T, Kimura K, Morita T (1995) Angiogenic therapy of acute myocardial infarction by intrapericardial injection of basic fibroblast growth factor and heparan sulfate: an experimental study. Am Heart J 130:1182–1188

Unger EF, Banai S, Shou M, Lazarous DF, Jaklitsch MT, Scheinowitz M, Correa R, Klingbeil C, Epstein SE (1994) Basic fibroblast growth factor enhances myocardial collateral flow in a canine model. Am J Physiol 266:H1588–1595

Ware JA, Simons M (1997) Angiogenesis in ischemic heart disease. Nat Med 3:158–164

Witmer-Pack MD, Hughes DA, Schuler G, Lawson L, McWilliam A, Inaba K, Steinman RM, Gordon S (1993) Identification of macrophages and dendritic cells in the osteopetrotic (op/op) mouse. J Cell Sci 104:1021–1029

Yanagisawa-Miwa A, Uchida Y, Nakamura F, Tomaru T, Kido H, Kamijo T, Sugimoto T, Kaji K, Utsuyama M, Kurashima C (1992) Salvage of infarcted myocardium by angiogenic action of basic fibroblast growth factor. Science 257:1401–1403

Zhou M, Sutliff RL, Paul RJ, Lorenz JN, Hoying JB, Haudenschild CC, Yin M, Coffin JD, Kong L, Kranias EG, Luo W, Boivin GP, Duffy JJ,

Pawlowski SA, Doetschman T (1998) Fibroblast growth factor 2 control of vascular tone. Nat Med 4:201–207

Ziche M, Morbidelli L, Masini E, Amerini S, Granger H, Maggi C, Geppetti P, Ledda F (1994) Nitric oxide medaites angiogenesis in vivo and endothelial cell growth and migration in vitro promoted by substance P. Am J Physiol 94:2036–2044

Ziche M, Morbidelli L, Choudhuri R, Zhang HT, Donnini S, Granger HJ, Bicknell R (1997) Nitric oxide synthase lies downstream from vascular endothelial growth factor-induced but not basic fibroblast growth factor-induced angiogenesis. J Clin Invest 99:2625–2634

8 Angiogenic Gene Therapy for Coronary Artery Disease

R.L. Engler

8.1 The Pathophysiology of Coronary Artery Disease as It Relates to Angiogenesis

An understanding of the basic morphology and pathophysiology of the coronary arteries is critical to understanding the interactive roles of gene therapy, bypass surgery, and angioplasty. Three principal vessels, branching off the left and right coronary ostea of the aorta, (the left anterior descending, circumflex, and right coronary arteries), serve the human heart. These vessels form a vascular tree with end capillary loops that generally do not interconnect (Factor et al. 1982). Thus, there are no native collateral vessels between major coronary arteries in the human heart. The pig is considered an excellent model for human coronary circulation, as it also has no native collateral vessels; whereas dogs have various, often extensive ones (Patterson and Kirk 1983). Nearly all ischemic heart disease is due to focal atherosclerotic narrowing of the large-surface coronary arteries. However, atherosclerosis tends to be a diffuse disease in the large epicardial coronary arteries; in it, some segments become narrowed from complex inflammatory and proliferative reactions (McPherson et al. 1992). Experimentally, the diffuse lipid deposits cluster at sites of low shear in larger vessels (100 μm); however, the locations where these deposits lead to atherosclerotic narrowing can not be predicted. Microcirculation is generally not affected by atherosclerotic narrowing. Syndromes involving defective microvascular dilation in response to metabolic need or shear can lead to ischemia, as well. Furthermore, hypercholesterolemia impairs shear-induced, nitric-oxide-dependent vasodilatation; an observation that may be relevant to angiogenesis because VEGF-induced angiogenesis is also nitric-oxide-dependent (Ziche et al. 1997; Sellke et al. 1990; Ohara et al. 1993; Fukai et al. 1998).

In response to repeated episodes of ischemia, collateral vessels form by angiogenesis. This process probably involves budding of new microvessels from existing capillaries, followed by progressive remodeling to form larger channels (Lewis et al. 1997; Zimmermann et al. 1997). When collateral formation is adequate during stress-induced increased myocardial oxygen demands, then the atherosclerotic disease will be asymptomatic. However, 7.5 million patients in the U.S. have symptomatic coronary artery disease. Some of these individuals have significant proximal stenosis of all three major coronary arteries, thus precluding effective collateral blood delivery. Collateral vessels originate far downstream in the microcirculation, generally from vessels less than 100 μm in size, and distal to the locations of atherosclerotic narrowing. In the majority of symptomatic patients, there is at least one adequate large vessel as a source of collaterals, yet they have angina. It appears that collateral formation stops short of complete relief of ischemia. Why the natural biologic process of angiogenesis in response to ischemia ceases is not at all known and is an important area for future research. The signal pathways that trigger the angiogenic response are under investigation. Preliminary studies indicate that induction of angiogenic growth factors such as vascular endothelial growth factor (VEGF) are initially increased but decrease over time in response to hypoxia.

Understanding the mechanism of premature cessation of angiogenesis may lead to specific mechanistic therapy.

A number of studies indicate that the natural angiogenic process can be enhanced or augmented. Reviewed elsewhere in this volume is evidence that protein therapy in a dog ameroid model of myocardial ischemia can speed collateral formation (Lazarous et al. 1996). However, the dog model has a number of infidelities with chronic myocardial ischemia in man. Dogs have native collaterals. An equally important biologic difference is that dogs, in response to ameroid coronary occlusion, continue to form collaterals for months until ischemia is completely relieved (Shou et al. 1997). In pigs, as in patients with angina, collateral development falls short of relieving ischemia during stress, even after 4 months (Roth et al. 1987).

8.2 Ameroid Model of Chronic Myocardial Ischemia

Abrupt occlusion of a coronary artery in the absence of pre-existing collaterals will result in acute myocardial infarction. In pigs, gradual occlusion of the artery over 7 to 14 days is accompanied by rapid development of collateral vessels and less than 2% infarction of the at-risk vascular bed (Roth et al. 1987, 1990). Gradual occlusion is accomplished by surgically placing an ameroid constrictor consisting of a "C" shaped steel ring surrounding a "C" shaped casine material around a coronary artery. This hygroscopic material gradually swells and is forced to expand inward by the steel ring to occlude the vessel. Pigs instrumented with ameroid constrictors have collateral-dependent myocardium distal to the occlusion. The collateral vessels function adequately at rest and there is no ischemia. However, during stress such as feeding, treadmill exercise, or rapid atrial pacing, the collateral-dependent myocardium becomes ischemic. This condition remains stable for at least 6 months, with no further evidence of collateral formation.

In the laboratories of Dr. Kirk Hammond at the VA San Diego Healthcare System, the pig ameroid model has been used to study angiogenic gene therapy (Giordano et al. 1996). Under general anesthesia, the ameroid constrictor is placed on the circumflex coronary artery along with a left atrial catheter and atrial pacing leads. Animals are allowed to recover for about 30 days and then are tested for stress-induced ischemia. Conscious animals supported in a sling are paced at twice the resting heart rate to a rate of about 200 bpm. A transthoracic echo is obtained prior to and during rapid atrial pacing. Wall thickening in the normally perfused LAD vascular bed and the collateral dependent circumflex bed is calculated by percentage. Normal wall thickening is about 65% at rest in the normally perfused LAD and collateral dependent circumflex beds. During rapid atrial pacing, thickening in the circumflex territory decreases by 50% or more due to myocardial ischemia. Animals that do not show adequate pacing-induced dysfunction are excluded from the protocol. Coronary flow is measured by contrast echo. Levovist (Berlex Labs) is injected through the left atrial catheter during continuous echo recording of the short axis view. The peak echo contrast ratio between the circumflex and LAD territories is an estimate of the flow ratio, validated by previous microsphere flow measurements. The flow ratio decreases by 50% or more during rapid atrial pacing, because flow increases in the normally perfused LAD bed but cannot increase as much in the collateral dependent territory. These animals show stable stress-induced ischemia for up to 6 months, the longest they have been followed. This model has been used to study the effect of angiogenic gene therapy on myocardial ischemia.

8.3 Adenoviral Vector Production

Human adenovirus serotype 5 (Ad5), rendered replication-incompetent by deletion of the E1A and E1B genes, was used. The CMV promoter and the cDNA for the gene to be studied linked to a polyadenylation tail was inserted into the deletion site (Giordano et al. 1996).

8.4 Initial Results: Gene Transfer with FGF-5

The fibroblast growth factor family consists of a number of alternately sliced and mutant genes coding for protcins that stimulate the FGF receptor family. There are four receptors with widespread expression in a large number of cell types. Activation of the receptors results in mitogenic activation through a variety of tyrosine kinase signaling pathways. One of the effects of FGF growth factors is angiogenesis.

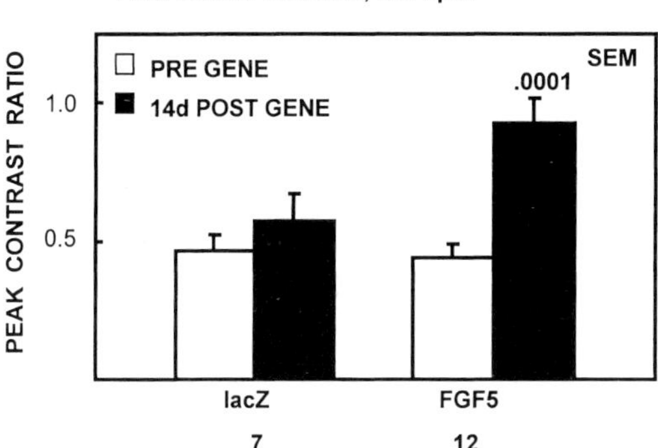

Fig. 1. Peak contrast ratio (by echocardiographic pixel intensity) between the left circumflex and left anterior descending beds represents the flow ratio. Normal intensity ratio is about 1.0 with this technique. The number below indicates the number of animals. *lacZ*, human adenovirus 5 with lacZ insert; *FGF5*, FGF5 cDNA insert; *pre-gene*, about 30 days after ameroid placement on left circumflex coronary artery (LCx)

In the chronic ameroid pig model, the first gene to be tested was FGF-5 (Giordano et al. 1996). Intracoronary injection of Ad5 with the insertion of the cDNA for either FGF-5 (Ad5-FGF5) or for β-galactosidase (Ad5-lacZ), as a control, was performed about 30 days after ameroid placement. Baseline flow and function by echocardiography was determined prior to gene transfer. Flow and function were again assessed 14 days after gene transfer. Analysis of the data was performed by individuals blinded to the treatment group. Gene transfer resulted in complete normalization of function and flow during pacing-induced stress in Ad5-FGF5-treated animals, but no significant change in Ad5-lacZ-treated control animals (Figs. 1, 2). An additional group of animals was followed for 12 weeks after gene transfer to ascertain if the improved flow and function would be sustained. There was no decline in the flow and function during stress between 2 and 12 weeks in Ad5-FGF5-treated animals.

Several important questions were further addressed in these initial studies:

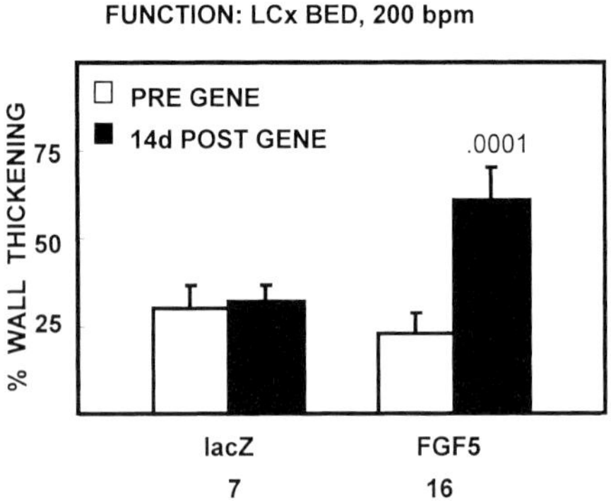

FUNCTION: LCx BED, 200 bpm

	PRE GENE	14d POST GENE
lacZ 7		
FGF5 16		.0001

% WALL THICKENING (25, 50, 75)

Fig. 2. Regional wall thickening in the left circumflex bed. Same groups of animals as in Fig. 1. *Pre-gene*, about 30 days after ameroid placement on left circumflex coronary artery; *14 days post-gene*, 14 days after intracoronary delivery of the adenovirus

1. Would the intracoronary delivery of adenovirus result in myocardial inflammation? Previous studies of direct intramyocardial injection of adenovirus found significant local inflammation in the area of the needle tract, associated with loss of gene expression within 7 weeks. In contrast, histologic sections of myocardium from intracoronarily injected hearts showed no evidence of inflammation at 2 or 12 weeks after treatment. Porcine specific anti-CD4 and anti-CD8 antibody staining demonstrated no T lymphocyte infiltration of the myocardium at 2 weeks post injection of adenovirus.
2. What is the extent of extracardiac gene transfer? One surprising result of this study was the observation of high first pass uptake of the virus by the myocardium. Blood was withdrawn from the pulmonary artery during Ad5-FGF5 injection and assayed for plaque-forming units. Using standard indicator dilution techniques to calculate the expected integrated pulmonary artery recovery of Ad5, the first pass extraction of Ad5 was found to be 98% upon intracoronary injection. When the residual amount of virus entering the pulmonary artery is diluted in the blood and delivered to the systemic circulation, the number of viral particles is extremely small relative to the total number of cells. It is well-established that ade-

novirus gene transfer and direct toxicity are dependent on the multiplicity of infection (MOI), or of transfection-competent viral particles per cell. There is about one transfection-competent (plaque forming unit, or PFU) per 100 viral particles. Gene transfection and expression generally require at least 10 PFU/cell. Thus, effective transfection of other organs would not be expected because the estimated PFU is much less than 1 PFU/1000 cells. Direct cytotoxicity from replication-incompetent adenovirus occurs at about 1000:1 MOI (>1000 PFU/cell). In this and subsequent studies (see below), tissue was harvested from liver, skeletal muscle, retina, and other organs. Gene transfer, gene transcription, and/or translation was tested by reverse transcriptase PCR, PCR, and/or immunoblot in these and subsequent experiments. Extracardiac gene expression generally has not been seen with successful intracoronary injection. Furthermore, gene transfer was below the sensitivity of the PCR assay for adenovirus (sensitivity of 10^4 viral particles/mg of tissue) in several key target organs: liver, kidney, retina, and skeletal muscle. In one lacZ animal, the injection was inadvertently made into the aorta, and gene transfer to liver was observed by β-galactosidase staining. Following left ventricular injection of 10^{12} viral particles, transgenic DNA was detected in testis 5 days after injection in one animal, but absent at 4 and 12 weeks. Lung tissue was positive by PCR but not by immunoblot after intracoronary delivery at the highest dose of 10^{12} viral particles. These results reflect the marked dilution of adenovirus after intracoronary delivery to MOI levels too low for efficient gene transfer. Previous studies of larger intraperitoneal or intravenous doses of adenovirus in rats showed evidence of liver inflammation. These findings may reflect the much higher MOI delivered.

3. Is the transgene expressed in the myocardium after gene transfer? Isolated cardiomyocytes transfected with Ad5-FGF5 secrete abundant FGF5 protein. Myocardial samples from porcine hearts in the Ad5-FGF5-treated group displayed mRNA for FGF5, and immunoblots showed abundant protein expression. Control Ad5-lacZ-treated animals did not demonstrate transgene message or protein production.
4. What is the mechanism of relief of myocardial ischemia in these studies? Hearts from several animals were subjected to rigorous his-

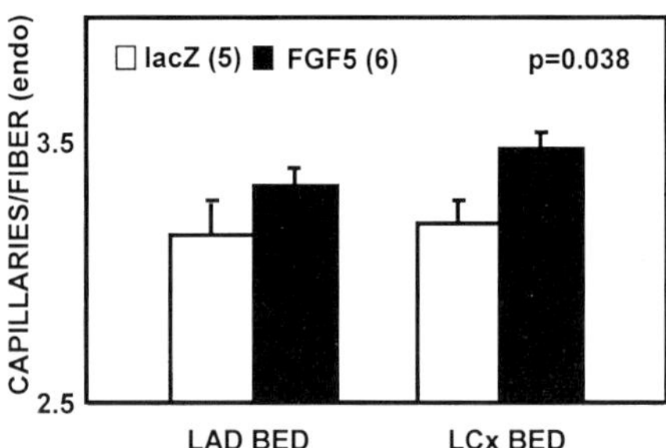

Fig. 3. Capillary:fiber ratio in Ad5-lacZ and Ad5-FGF5-treated animals (vessels <10 μm). Hearts were perfusion-fixed at constant pressure. There was also an increase in larger vessels (>10 μm) only in the circumflex bed, but the number of hearts available was only three from each group

tologic analysis. Defined pressure perfusion fixation was performed and tissue blocks were obtained from the collateral-dependent circumflex and the normal LAD bed. The capillary to fiber ratio (microvessels <10 μm in diameter) was determined by observers blinded to treatment group and sample site. There was a significant increase in capillary:fiber ratio in the microcirculation of Ad5-FGF5-treated animals (Fig. 3). Only three hearts could be examined for larger vessels, due to different sectioning requirements for this type of analysis. There was an increase in larger vessels only in the circumflex bed, but the number of animals was too small for statistical analysis. These results indicate that the mechanism of relief of myocardial ischemia was angiogenesis, improving collateral blood flow.

5. Experiments conducted with a genetically engineered mutant of bFGF with and without a signal peptide indicate that secretion is necessary for an angiogenic response sufficient to relieve ischemia. These experiments also serve to confirm the lacZ control findings that relief of ischemia is dependent on FGF production and receptor stimulation, and not a consequence of the adenovirus per se.

In summary, these experiments showed that intracoronary adenoviral vector injection results in high-efficiency gene transfer to the myocardium, and that doses of up to 5×10^{11} viral particles will not result in significant systemic gene transfer at the sensitivity level of detection used in these studies. Transfection of FGF5 and several other FGF angiogenic genes can augment endogenous collateral formation sufficient to relieve myocardial ischemia.

8.5 Other Angiogenic Genes

Published studies have used a number of other angiogenic genes and proteins in the pig or dog ameroid model. The two classes of genes that have been tested are FGFs and VEGFs. Recently, hepatocyte growth factor and neuropeptide Y have also shown promise as angiogenic genes (Van Belle et al. 1998; Ono et al. 1997; Zukowska-Grojec et al. 1998). FGFs are a family of related proteins that stimulate FGF receptors. Most are bound with high affinity to the glycocalyx through heparin binding characteristics. The two prototypes are acidic FGF (aFGF, FGF-1) and basic FGF (bFGF, FGF-2). Acidic and basic FGF are not secreted by the classic Golgi pathway. Instead, FGF-1 and FGF-2 are exported by a recently discovered novel secretory pathway (Tarantini et al. 1995; Maciag and Friesel 1995). Both VEGF and FGF proteins (i.e., not gene therapy) have been shown to be angiogenic in animal models (Lazarous et al. 1996; Banai et al. 1994; Pearlman et al. 1995; Harada et al. 1994). The vascular endothelial growth factor (VEGF) family consists of four genes (VEGF-A, VEGF-B, VEGF-C, and VEGF-D), with several splice variants for VEGF-A. These gene products are mostly endothelial-cell-specific, being mitogenic through stimulation of three receptors, FLT-1, FLK-1, and FLT-4 (Keyt et al. 1996), although VEGF-A-165 also affects monocytes and macrophages. VEGF-induced angiogenesis is dependent on nitric oxide, but bFGF angiogenesis is not (Ziche et al. 1997).

Direct intramyocardial injection of aFGF has been shown to enhance native angiogenesis after coronary artery bypass surgery in patients with nonrevascularized regions (Schumacher et al. 1998). Direct epicardial injections resulted in enhanced microvascular flow visible by angiography. This randomized, blinded trial gives proof of the principle that natural angiogenesis can be enhanced in patients with ischemic heart disease.

In porcine studies, a mutant FGF-2 gene constructed by insertion of a short segment of the interlukin-1 gene engineered with a signal peptide, also relieved ischemia at equivalent viral particle doses. However, when the secretory signal peptide was omitted, the effects were markedly reduced or absent at the same dose of virus. This result suggests that secretion, in this case through the classic Golgi pathway to export the protein into the interstitium of the heart, enhances the angiogenic effect. However, full dose-response relationships were not determined, so the absolute importance of secretion cannot be assessed at the current time.

8.6 The Role of FGF-4

FGF-4 is an angiogenic, mitogenic gene normally only expressed during fetal development. Experiments in the Hammond lab found that Ad5-FGF4 was as efficacious as Ad5-FGF5 in relieving myocardial ischemia at roughly equivalent doses of viral particles. A dose-response curve identified the minimal effective dose that resulted in relief of ischemia (unpublished data).

A combined phase I and II clinical trial in patients with chronic stable angina was initiated based on these preclinical experiments and additional toxicology studies. Patients with chronic stable angina, class 2 or 3, are enrolled for intracoronary delivery of Ad5-FGF4. The placebo control is saline, which was chosen for the safety aspects of the study. Animal trials have been adequately performed and have found a lack of angiogenic effects from replication-incompetent adenovirus. The endpoints of the trial are treadmill exercise and dobutamine stress echocardiography.

8.7 Other Routes for Gene Therapy

Intrapericardial administration of adenovirus with a marker gene has been studied (Lamping et al. 1997). Transfection efficiency was confined to the first few cell layers of the visceral and parietal pericardium and only occasionally was detected in epicardial myocytes. Intrapericardial injection of hemoglutinating virus of Japan (HVJ) liposomes to transfect marker DNA after injection shows somewhat more efficient gene transfer (Aoki et al. 1997). These techniques have potential as a route for delivery of gene therapy to the epicardium of the heart. However, transfection efficiency appears to be limited. Direct injection of bFGF protein into the pericardial space of dogs failed to produce sufficient angiogenesis to relieve myocardial ischemia in the ameroid model. Taken together, these findings suggest that the pericardial route of administering gene therapy for angiogenesis is not likely to be successful; however, no direct test has been published.

Direct myocardial injection of adenovirus results in significant transfection near the needle track, but is associated with inflammation. This method has been used to transfect myocardium with marker genes and VEGF (Magovern et al. 1996). Preliminary studies in the pig ameroid model indicated relief of myocardial ischemia (unpublished results). A clinical trial has been initiated for intramyocardial injection of adenovirus with $VEGF_{121}$ at the time of coronary artery bypass graft surgery to augment angiogenesis in areas nonamenable to bypass.

8.8 Transmyocardial Laser Revascularization

No discussion of angiogenic therapy would be complete without mention of transmyocardial (TMR) or endocardial laser revascularization. Application of laser energy from either the epicardial surface at the time of thoracotomy or on the endocardial surface has been shown to engender a local angiogenic response associated with increased production of bFGF and transforming growth factor beta around the site of injury. These results were observed when the injury was induced with a needle (Pelletier et al. 1998). Following TMR or endocardial laser the "channels" created do not stay open. Thus, the mechanism of relief of ischemia using laser revascularization is an angiogenic response to injury. TMR has been found to augment maximal blood flow to the area of the occluded left anterior descending coronary artery in the dog model (Yamamoto et al. 1998). It has been proposed that laser revascularization might be augmented by the addition of angiogenic growth factors. In a pig model of transmyocardial laser revascularization, the addition of VEGF or adenovirus coding the human profilin gene increased nonspecific histologic response to injury and inflammation but resulted in no additional angiogenesis (Fleischer et al. 1996). The potential for augmenting angiogenesis in response to laser revascularization needs further clinical evaluation.

As an adjunct to coronary artery bypass graft surgery, transmyocardial laser revascularization has recently been approved for patients with severe, refractory ischemia not amenable to surgical revascularization. The relatively invasive nature of laser revascularization, and concomitant trauma and inflammation to the myocardium are significant limitations of this technique. Furthermore, newer developments in angiogenesis techniques may improve or replace this surgical procedure.

8.9 Conclusion

We can be reasonably optimistic that angiogenic therapy will be available for patients with coronary artery disease in the near future. Studies in the porcine model of chronic myocardial ischemia, in which natural angiogenesis shuts off prior to relief of ischemia, clearly demonstrates the ability to augment the angiogenic process. A number of experimental studies using protein delivery by epicardial beads or intracoronary administration indicate the feasibility of augmenting angiogenesis. In humans, a blinded, randomized placebo-controlled clinical trial with aFGF protein provides proof of this principle. A number of clinical trials are underway to sort out the optimum route of delivery of genes or proteins to be utilized. Herein, we have not reviewed protein angiogenic therapy; however, suffice it to say that, based on animal studies, repeated administration will probably be necessary. If gene therapy with angiogenic growth factors proves successful, single administration will likely replace any developments in protein angiogenesis therapy. Routes of administration for gene therapy under clinical development include intracoronary adenovirus and direct epicardial injection of adenovirus. Depending on clinical circumstances, several different modes of therapy might be valuable tools for the invasive cardiologist and/or cardiac surgeon.

References

Aoki M, Morishita R, Muraishi A, Moriguchi A, Sugimoto T, Maeda K, Dzau VJ, Kaneda Y, Higaki J, Ogihara T (1997) Efficient in vivo gene transfer into the heart in the rat myocardial infarction model using the HVJ (hemagglutinating virus of Japan)–liposome method. J Mol Cell Cardiol 29:949–959

Banai S, Jaklitsch MT, Shou M, Lazarous D. F, Scheinowitz M, Biro S, Epstein SE, Unger EF (1994) Angiogenic-induced enhancement of collateral blood flow to ischemic myocardium by vascular endothelial growth factor in dogs. Circulation 89:2183–2189

Factor SM, Okun EM, Minase T, Kirk ES (1982) The microcirculation of the human heart: end-capillary loops with discrete perfusion fields. The microcirculation of the human heart: end-capillary loops with discrete perfusion fields. Circulation 66:1241–1248

Fleischer KJ, Goldschmidt-Clermont PJ, Fonger JD, Hutchins GM, Hruban RH, Baumgartner WA (1996) One-month histologic response of transmyocardial laser channels with molecular intervention. Ann Thorac Surg 62:1051–1058

Fukai T, Galis ZS, Meng XP, Parthasarathy S, Harrison DG (1998) Vascular expression of extracellular superoxide dismutase in atherosclerosis. J Clin Invest 101:2101–2111

Giordano FJ, Ping P, McKirnan MD, Nozaki S, DeMaria AN, Dillmann WH, Mathieu-Costello O, Hammond HK (1996) Intracoronary gene transfer of fibroblast growth factor-5 increases blood flow and contractile function in an ischemic region of the heart (see comments). Nat Med 2:534–539

Harada K, Grossman W, Friedman M, Edelman ER, Prasad PV, Keighley CS, Manning WJ, Sellke FW, Simons M (1994) Basic fibroblast growth factor improves myocardial function in chronically ischemic porcine hearts. J Clin Invest 94:623–630

Keyt BA, Nguyen HV, Berleau LT, Duarte CM, Park J, Chen H, and Ferrara N (1996) Identification of vascular endothelial growth factor determinants for binding KDR and FLT-1 receptors. Generation of receptor-selective VEGF variants by site-directed mutagenesis. J Biol Chem 271:5638–5646

Lamping KG, Rios CD, Chun JA, Ooboshi H, Davidson BL, Heistad DD (1997) Intrapericardial administration of adenovirus for gene transfer. Am J Physiol 272:H310–317

Lazarous DF, Shou M, Scheinowitz M, Hodge E, Thirumurti V, Kitsiou AN, Stiber JA, Lobo AD, Hunsberger S, Guetta E, Epstein SE, Unger EF (1996) Comparative effects of basic fibroblast growth factor and vascular endothelial growth factor on coronary collateral development and the arterial response to injury. Circulation 94:1074–1082

Lewis BS, Flugelman MY, Weisz A, Keren-Tal I, Schaper W (1997) Angiogenesis by gene therapy: a new horizon for myocardial revascularization? Cardiovasc Res 35:490–497

Maciag T, Friesel RE (1995) Molecular mechanisms of fibroblast growth factor-1 trafficking, signaling and release. Thromb Haemost 74:411–414

Magovern CJ, Mack CA, Zhang J, Hahn RT, Ko W, Isom OW, Crystal RG, Rosengart TK (1996) Direct in vivo gene transfer to canine myocardium using a replication-deficient adenovirus vector. Ann Thorac Surg 62:425–433; discussion 433–434

McPherson DD, Johnson MR, Alvarez NM, Rewcastle NB, Collins SM, Armstrong ML, Kieso RA, Thorpe LJ, Marcus ML, Kerber RE (1992) Variable morphology of coronary atherosclerosis: characterization of atherosclerotic plaque and residual arterial lumen size and shape by epicardial echocardiography. J Am Coll Cardiol 19:593–599

Ohara Y, Peterson TE, Harrison DG (1993) Hypercholesterolemia increases endothelial superoxide anion production. J Clin Invest 91:2546–2551

Ono K, Matsumori A, Shioi T, Furukawa Y, Sasayama S (1997) Enhanced expression of hepatocyte growth factor/c-met by myocardial ischemia and reperfusion in a rat model (see comments). Circulation 95:2552–2558

Patterson RE, Kirk ES (1983) Analysis of coronary collateral structure, function, and ischemic border zones in pigs. Am J Physiol 244:H23–31

Pearlman JD, Hibberd MG, Chuang ML, Harada K, Lopez JJ, Gladstone SR, Friedman M, Sellke FW, Simons M (1995) Magnetic resonance mapping demonstrates benefits of VEGF-induced myocardial angiogenesis (see comments). Nat Med 1:1085–1089

Pelletier MP, Giaid A, Sivaraman S, Dorfman J, Li CM, Philip A, Chiu RC (1998) Angiogenesis and growth factor expression in a model of transmyocardial revascularization. Ann Thorac Surg 66:12–18

Roth DM, White FC, Nichols ML, Dobbs SL, Longhurst JC, Bloor CM (1990) Effect of long-term exercise on regional myocardial function and coronary collateral development after gradual coronary artery occlusion in pigs. Circulation 82:1778–1789

Roth DM, Maruoka Y, Rogers J, White FC, Longhurst JC, Bloor CM (1987) Development of coronary collateral circulation in left circumflex ameroid-occluded swine myocardium. Am J Physiol 253:H1279–1288

Schumacher B, Pecher P, von Specht BU, Stegmann T (1998) Induction of neoangiogenesis in ischemic myocardium by human growth factors: first clinical results of a new treatment of coronary heart disease (see comments). Circulation 97:645–650

Sellke FW, Armstrong ML, Harrison DG (1990) Endothelium-dependent vascular relaxation is abnormal in the coronary microcirculation of atherosclerotic primates. Circulation 81:1586–1593

Shou M, Thirumurti V, Rajanayagam S, Lazarous DF, Hodge E, Stiber JA, Pettiford M, Elliott E, Shah SM, Unger EF (1997) Effect of basic fibroblast growth factor on myocardial angiogenesis in dogs with mature collateral vessels (see comments). J Am Coll Cardiol 29:1102–1106

Tarantini F, Gamble S, Jackson A, Maciag T (1995) The cysteine residue responsible for the release of fibroblast growth factor-1 residues in a domain independent of the domain for phosphatidylserine binding. J Biol Chem 270:29039–29042

Van Belle E, Witzenbichler B, Chen D, Silver M, Chang L, Schwall R, Isner JM (1998) Potentiated angiogenic effect of scatter factor/hepatocyte growth factor via induction of vascular endothelial growth factor: the case for paracrine amplification of angiogenesis. Circulation 97:381–390

Yamamoto N, Kohmoto T, Gu A, DeRosa C, Smith CR, Burkhoff D (1998) Angiogenesis is enhanced in ischemic canine myocardium by transmyocardial laser revascularization. J Am Coll Cardiol 31:1426–1433

Ziche M, Morbidelli L, Choudhuri R, Zhang HT, Donnini S, Granger HJ, Bicknell R (1997) Nitric oxide synthase lies downstream from vascular endothelial growth factor-induced but not basic fibroblast growth factor-induced angiogenesis. J Clin Invest 99:2625–2634

Zimmermann R, Arras M, Ullmann C, Strasser R, Sack S, Mollnau H, Schaper J, Schaper W (1997) Time course of mitosis and collateral growth following coronary microembolization in the porcine heart. Cell Tissue Res 287:583–590

Zukowska-Grojec Z, Karwatowska-Prokopczuk E, Rose W, Rone J, Movafagh S, Ji H, Yeh Y, Chen WT, Kleinman HK, Grouzmann E, Grant DS (1998) Neuropeptide Y: a novel angiogenic factor from the sympathetic nerves and endothelium. Circ Res 83:187–195

9 Transmyocardial Laser Use for Endstage Coronary Artery Disease

S.F. Aranki, F. Mannting, S.K. Shernan, N.C. Cummings,
S.P. Sears, L.H. Cohn

9.1 Introduction

Transmyocardial laser revascularization (TMLR) is a relatively new treatment modality for patients with inoperable end stage coronary artery disease. It results in significant relief of angina in patients with end-stage coronary artery disease. The indications for this therapy are still evolving as results of ongoing and recently completed studies are extensively scrutinized. Continuous evaluation is essential in order to verify the validity of these results and establish long-term outcomes. The objective of this report is to analyze our data for 53 TMLR procedures performed over the last 5 years.

9.2 Evaluation of Myocardial Revascularization

Attempts at indirect myocardial revascularization preceded the era of modern cardiac surgery ushered in by the introduction of the cardiopulmonary bypass by Gibbon (Gibbon 1939). The most famous of these indirect procedures was the Vineberg procedure (Vineberg 1954), which would have been the standard means of myocardial revascularization, had it not been eclipsed by the introduction of coronary artery bypass graft surgery (CABG) by Favaloro (Favaloro 1968). This was made possible by the introduction of selective coronary angioplasty by Sones (Sones and Shirey 1962). Direct myocardial revascularization represented by CABG and percutaneous transluminal coronary angioplasty (PTCA) are currently the gold standard for myocardial revascularization. They continue to evolve with the employment of more arterial conduits and better stent designs.

Paradoxically, in spite of the major advances in the treatment of atherosclerotic coronary artery disease (CAD) over the last 30 years, there is an emerging group of patients with advanced and inoperable disease. These patients have had multiple surgical or interventional procedures in the past to treat their CAD. The arteries are small, diffusely diseased, and even coronary endarterectomy is not an option. Such patients usually have advanced symptomatic angina and a miserable existence with a poor quality of life.

The use ofTMLR was introduced by Mirhoseini et al. (1988; Mirhoseini and Dayton 1981) in order to create transmyocardial channels extending from the epicardial surface of the free wall of the left ventricle to the left ventricular chamber. The rationale was to supply blood directly to the left ventricular myocardium through these channels, that were thought to stay open permanently. Further experimental and clinical studies have failed to decipher the exact mechanisms of action of TMLR.

9.3 Study Report

9.3.1 Materials and Methods

The Brigham and Women's Hospital was a participant in phase II and phase III studies by the U.S. Food and Drug Administration. Phase II was a nonrandomized prospective trial involving 201 patients at eight U.S. clinical centers. The aim of the study was to establish the degrees of safety, efficacy, and utility of TMLR. Phase III study, involving 197 patients, was a prospective randomized study to confirm the results of phase II study and compare TMLR with continued maximal medical therapy.

9.3.1.1 Patients

Between March 1993 and September 1998, 53 patients underwent TMLR at the Brigham and Women's Hospital. Informed consent was obtained from all patients. The inclusion criteria were refractory class 3 or 4 CSS angina (Canadian Cardiovascular Society), reversible ischemia in the free wall of the left ventricle, and the presence of coronary arteries that were not suitable for CABG or PTCA. Patients with an ejection fraction <20% and those with concurrent, severe illness were excluded from the study.

The patients were followed up at 3, 6, and 12 month intervals. Angina class, quality of life questionnaires, and nuclear scans were compared at these intervals to corresponding preoperative studies.

9.3.1.2 Operative Procedure

General anesthesia with a double lumen endotracheal tube is similar to that in other cardiac surgical procedures. A combination of narcotics, barbiturates, and muscle relaxants is used for induction. Maintenance of anesthesia is achieved with volatile inhalation agents supplemented by further narcotics, as necessary. Hemodynamic monitoring is achieved with a radial arterial line and a pulmonary artery catheter. In addition, transesophageal echocardiography (TEE) is essential for hemodynamic monitoring, detection of myocardial ischemia, confirming the transmyocardial penetration of the laser channels, and to check for injury to the mitral valve apparatus.

Because of the severe, advanced nature of CAD and the fact that relief of ischemia is not instantaneous, TMLR patients are extremely fragile. Acute ischemia and compromised hemodynamics may develop rapidly. Consequently, acute myocardial infarction and cardiogenic shock are most likely to result in an unfavorable outcome. Therefore, intravenous nitrates are used routinely in most patients undergoing TMLR, as is intravenous heparin in the intensive care unit after the risk of bleeding has abated.

Mechanical support is provided by the prophylactic insertion of a percutaneous intra-aortic balloon pump (IABP) in the operating room before starting the surgical procedure. This has been used routinely in our last 23 patients. Our prior experience indicated that postoperative insertion of an IABP in the intensive care unit usually came too late to be of any benefit. Intravenous heparin, nitrates, and use of the IABP are continued for at least 48 h postoperatively. However, hemodynamically stable patients could be extubated as early as possible.

The operation is performed through a lateral thoracotomy, with the patient lying supine and on the left side. The left pleural cavity is entered through the fourth or fifth intercostal space. Lung isolation with a double lumen tube allows for collapse of the left lung. This is essential for better exposure and division of scar tissue between the lung, chest wall, and pericardium, since an overwhelming majority of the patients had already had one or more CABG procedures.

The pericardium is opened above and in a parallel fashion to the left phrenic nerve. Thick pericardial adhesions between the pericardium and the underlying epicardial surface of the left ventricle are carefully divided where the free wall of the left ventricle is freed from the overlying pericardium. The areas of the left ventricular free wall that were predesignated by use of nuclear scans as being under risk for ischemia are targeted primarily for the creation of the laser channels. Because angiogenesis is believed to be the likely mechanism of action, we now target nonischemic areas, as well.

9.3.1.3 The Laser Device

The laser channels are created by a high powered carbon dioxide laser. (The CO_2 Heart Laser System, PLC Medical Systems, Franklin, Mass.). This can deliver 850 W of peak power to the myocardial tissues. A holmium-neon laser guide is used to aim the CO_2 laser beam at the epicardium of the left ventricular free wall. The laser is synchronized with the electrocardiogram and triggered to coincide with the R wave. The channels are confirmed by TEE when the laser energy is absorbed by the blood in the left ventricular cavity. A 1 mm channel is created, resulting in one channel per cm^2 of epicardial surface. Bleeding from these channels is easily controlled with digital compression.

9.3.2 Results

The preoperative characteristics are summarized in Table 1; the frequency of risk factors and comorbid conditions for CAD patients are shown in Table 2. The striking feature of this patient population is that 89% had previously undergone a CABG. This is indicative of the longstanding, advanced nature of CAD in these patients. It is also noticeable that almost half the patients are diabetic, attesting to the severity and diffuse nature of CAD.

9.3.3 Operative Variables

There was an average of 26 channels (with a range of 11–46), confirmed by TEE. Hemostasis was successfully achieved with digital compression in well over 99% of the patients. One patient with a patent vein graft to the marginal branch of the circumflex artery suffered abrupt occlusion of the vein graft and required emergency cardiac catheterization, and the vein graft was reopened. The mean ICU stay was 2.7±1 days, and 30% of all patients stayed longer than 10 days in the hospital.

9.3.4 Mortality

There were no intraoperative deaths in this patient group. A total of seven patients died within 30 days (13%). Four of these deaths occurred among phase II patients and three among phase III patients. There was only one perioperative death (within 30 days) among the last 23 patients, in whom we routinely initiated intra-aortic balloon counterpulsa-

Table 1. Baseline patient characteristics and demographics

Age	46–84 years; mean 63.1 years; 21% over 70 years
Sex	42 males (79%); 11 females (21%)
Angina class	43% class III; 57% class IV
Prior CABG	47 (89%)
Prior PTCA	16 (30%)
Ejection fraction	20–71%; mean 48%
Prior Myocardial infarction	40 (70%)
Congestive heart failure	13 (25%)

Table 2. Cardiac risk factors and associated comorbidities

Risk factors	Number of patients (percentage)
Hypertension	37 (70%)
Diabetes	27 (50%)
Hypercholesterolemia	33 (62%)
Smoking history	37 (70%)
Family history	26 (49%)
Peripheral vascular disease	9 (17%)
Transient ischemic attack	4 (8%)
Cerebrovascular accident	6 (11%)
Carotid endarterectomy	4 (8%)
Chronic obstructive pulmonary disease	11 (25%)

tion prior to starting operative procedure. In six patients, the causes of death were cardiac-related. One patient died from acute hypotension related to epidural narcotic overdose.

During the follow-up period (100% complete; range of 3–65 months; mean of 25 months), 12 patients died between 37 days and 59 months postoperatively. Causes of late death were cardiac in eight patients, noncardiac in three, and accidental in one. The overall survival rate at 24 months' follow-up was 64%. Multivariate analysis identified age above 65 years an independent predictor of death as was the presence of peripheral vascular disease.

During follow-up, six patients required PCTA stent of previously patent vein grafts or because of progression of native CAD; one required CABG due to occlusion of a previously patent vein graft; one required a subsequent TMLR procedure; and one required mitral valve replacement 37 months after the initial surgery, due to papillary muscle rupture.

9.3.5 Angina Class

A decline of two angina classes following TMLR was considered a success. The median angina class was reduced from four preoperatively to two at 3 months, and to one at 6 and 12 months, respectively. Whereas 100% of the patients were in class 3 or 4 prior to surgery, only 8%, 6%, and 4% were in this category at 3, 6, and 12 months follow-up, respectively ($p<0.005$).

Medications used to treat CAD were recorded before and at 3, 6, and 12 month intervals following TMLR. The use of oral nitrates, beta blockers, and calcium channel blockers was mainly unchanged or slightly reduced to nonsignificant levels.

9.3.6 Nuclear Scans

Thallium-201 single positron omission tomography (^{201}TI:SPECT), with pharmacologic stress (dipyridamole) and 4 h re-injection with redistribution, was performed to assess the reversibility of myocardial ischemia. The extent of a perfusion abnormality was computed and expressed as percent of total myocardium volume. The severity of a perfusion abnormality in the angina sector is determined by the number of standard deviations the tracer uptake is below the lower limit of normal. Compared with the preoperative baseline data, our data showed that the extent and severity of stress-induced ischemia decreased postoperatively. However, this decrease reached only borderline statistical significance ($p=0.04$). The extent and severity of the rest perfusion abnormalities, which reflect scarring tended to also increase post operatively, reaching lower level statistical significance ($p<0.05$).

9.4 Discussion

TMLR is a relatively new treatment modality for advanced and inoperable CAD that is refractory to maximal medical therapy. Its exact mechanism of action remains unknown. However, it is certain that TMLR acts indirectly by providing new blood supply to the ischemic myocardium. Establishing new blood flow directly to the existing coronary arteries (with PTCA on CABG) is not possible, due to the severe and advanced nature of CAD.

The results of this study show the effectiveness of TMLR in relieving severe angina to a great extent, and thereby improving the quality of life. Because of the severity of CAD, these patients are liable to become ischemic under stressful conditions such as general anesthesia and major surgery such as TMLR – the likelihood of developing acute myocardial insufficiency, acute myocardial infarction, and cardiogenic shock are extremely high. In addition, TMLR does not cause instantaneous improvement in myocardial blood supply. Such improvement occurs gradually over a period of weeks or even months. Consequently, any intraoperative ischemia instability may continue with high probability of a bad outcome into the postoperative period. It is therefore essential that maximal pharmacological and mechanical support be instituted in the operating room prior to the operative procedure. Such prophylactic measures are certain to improve the perioperative outcome in this group of patients. Adjunctive use of hemodynamic monitoring and transesophageal echocardiography is also essential in detecting ischemia and confirming the response to the instituted therapy.

The results of this study are consistent with those of other reported studies on TMLR, as far as survival, relief of angina, and improved quality of life are concerned (Cooley et al. 1996; Frazier et al. 1995; Horvath et al. 1996, 1997; Vincent et al. 1997). However, the objective correlation of improved myocardial perfusion as represented by nuclear scans is somewhat weaker. This may be related either to the fact that these tests are not consistently reproducible or that the improvement in angina may not be related directly to improved myocardial perfusion alone. Therefore, this apparent discrepancy will continue until the exact mechanism of action of TMLR has been established.

The concept of creating transmyocardial channels is not new. Sen et al. (1965) reported on "transmyocardial acupuncture" by producing a direct communication between the left ventricular cavity and the myocardial sinuses. Other investigators reported similar attempts and documented improved blood flow through the myocardium (Hershey and White 1969; Walter et al. 1971). The rationale behind these attempts was based on the original work of Wearns et al. (1933), who reported on the existence of a micro vascular system consisting of an extensive network of sinusoids and capillaries. This network has a direct connection with the coronary arteries as well as the left ventricular cavity.

These early attempts at transmyocardial revascularization were overshadowed by the introduction of CABG and PTCA. However, the concept resurfaced with the emergence of a subset of patients with end-stage CAD in whom conventional methods of direct myocardial revascularization were not possible. Initial attempts with a low-powered laser were reported by Mirhoseini et al. (1988; Mirhoseini and Cayton 1981), who used it in conjunction with CABG surgery. The introduction of a high powered laser synchronized to the R wave of the electrocardiogram (The CO_2 Heart Laser System) made possible the creation of transmyocardial laser channels with minimal thermal damage and a markedly reduced incidence of ventricular arrhythmia. A phase I pilot study was conducted at the San Francisco Heart Institute which paved the way for the phase II and phase III trials sponsored by the FDA.

Several mechanisms of action of TMLR have been proposed. These include the placebo effect, myocardial damage and necrosis, myocardial denervation, direct blood supply through patent channels, and promotion and development of new blood supply (angiogenesis). Since angina relief takes a few weeks or months to develop, the placebo factor, the myocardial necrosis and denervation factors become highly unlikely mechanisms of action. In addition, the transmyocardial channels are unlikely to stay patent. Therefore, the angiogenesis theory represents the most plausible but by no means the only mechanism for angina relief (Gassler and Stubbe 1997). It is highly likely that a combination of the above factors are responsible at variable intervals and to various extents.

In summary, based on the results of this study, the important question is whether we should continue to offer this therapy to patients with end-stage coronary artery disease. Because of the marked improvements it can bring in angina severity and quality of life, many patients continue to choose this treatment option. Although the perioperative risks seem to be high, comparable to those associated with major cardiac surgery such as repeat CABG, we believe that instituting maximal pharmacological and mechanical support will significantly reduce the perioperative risk.

Other important questions relate to the long-term duration of angina relief and the impact of TMLR on long-term survival. The results so far (phase III report to the FDA) seem to indicate that long-term survival is comparable to that with continued medical therapy. However, the question of long-term freedom from angina remains to be established by study of longer-term follow-ups.

References

Cooley DA, Frazier OH, Kadipasaoglu KA, Lindenmeier MH, Pehlivanoglu S, Kolff JW, Wilansky S, Moore WH (1996) Transmyocardial laser revascularization: clinical experience with twelve-months follow-up. J Thorac Cardiovasc Surg 111:791–799

Favaloro RG (1968) Saphenous vein autograft replacement of severe segmental coronary artery occlusion: operative technique. Ann Thorac Surg 5:334–339

Frazier OH, Cooley DA, Kadipasaoglu KA et al. (1995) Myocardial revascularization with laser: preliminary findings. Circulation 92:II58–65

Gassler N, Stubbe HM (1997) Clinical data and histological features of transmyocardial revascularization with CO_2 laser. Eur J Cardiothorac Surg 12:25–30

Gibbon JH Jr (1939) The maintenance of life during experimental occlusion of the pulmonary artery followed by survival. Surg Gynecol Obstet 69:602

Hershey JE, White M (1969) Transmyocardial puncture revascularization: a possible emergency adjunct to arterial implant surgery. Geriatrics 24:101–108

Horvath KA, Cohn LH, Cooley DA, Crew JR, Frazier OH, Griffith BP, Kadipasaoglu K, Lansing A, Mannting F, March R, Mirhoseini MR, Craig S. (1997) Transmyocardial laser revascularization used as sole therapy for end-stage coronary artery disease. J Thorac Cardiovasc Surg 113:645–654

Horvath K, Mannting F, Cummings N et al. (1996) Transmyocardial laser revascularizatoin: operative techniques and clinical results at two years. J Thorac Cardiovasc Surg 111:1046–1053

Mirhoseini M, Cayton M (1981) Revascularizatoin of the heart by laser. J Microsurg 2:253–260

Mirhoseini M, Shelgikar S, Cayton M (1988) New concepts in revascularization of the myocardium. Ann Thorac Surg 45:415–420

Sen PK, Udwadia TE, Kinare SG, Parulkar GB (1965) Transmyocardial acupuncture. J Thorac Cardiovasc Surg 50:181–189

Sones FM Jr, Shirey EK (1962) Cine coronary arteriography. Mod Concepts Cardiovasc Dis 31:735–738

Vincent JG, Bardos P, Maass D (1997) End-stage coronary artery disease treated with the transmyocardial CO_2 laser revascularization: a chance for the inoperable patient. Eur J Carthorac Surg 11:888–894

Vineberg A (1954) Clinical and experimental studies in the treatment of coronary artery insufficiency by internal artery implant. J Int Coll Surg 22:503–518

Walter P, Hundeshagen H, Borst HG (1971) Treatment of acute myocardial infarction by transmural blood supply from the ventricular cavity. Eur Surg Res 3:130–138

Wearns JT, Mettier SR, Klump TG, Ziesche AB (1933) The nature of the vascular communications between the coronary arteries and the chambers of the heart. Am Heart J 9:143–170

10 Vascular Gene Therapy – Early Clinical Results with Angiogenic Growth Factors

S. Ylä-Herttuala

10.1 Introduction

Gene therapy offers an interesting alternative for the treatment of various inherited and acquired diseases. Treatment of restenosis and induction of therapeutic angiogenesis in ischemic tissues are among the first candidates for clinical gene therapy trials, since only temporary expression of the transgene is required for a therapeutic effect (Ylä-Herttuala 1997). Several candidate treatment genes are currently available for these conditions (see below), and recent developments in gene transfer and vector technology have also improved our ability to achieve clinically significant levels of transgene expression in vivo.

10.2 Gene Transfer Vectors

Naked plasmids, plasmid/liposomes and adenoviruses have been most widely used vectors in vascular gene transfer studies. Naked plasmids and plasmid/liposomes lead to transient expression with a relatively low transfection efficiency (Laitinen et al. 1997). However, they are easy to prepare and well-tolerated without any considerable danger. Adenoviruses also cause a transient transfection effect, but the level of expression achieved in transfected tissues is much higher (Laitinen et al. 1997). Intravascular gene transfer has generally produced lower transfection efficiencies than intramuscular gene transfer has (Isner et al. 1996). Retroviruses have also been widely used in gene transfer studies. However, they have not been used for cardiovascular applications, since transfection efficiency with retroviruses is low (Laitinen et al. 1997) and stable transfection is not needed in cardiovascular applications.

10.3 Angiogenic Factors

The vascular endothelial growth factor (VEGF) has been the most widely used factor for therapeutic angiogenesis (Isner 1997). The VEGF family has several members: VEGF-A, VEGF-B, VEGF-C, VEGF-D, VEGF-E, and the placental growth factor (Korpelainen and Alitalo 1998). VEGF-A also has several isoforms generated through alternative splicing: VEGF-121, VEGF-145, VEGF-165, VEGF-189, and VEGF-206 (Ferrara and Buntling 1996). In animal experiments, VEGF-121, VEGF-165, and VEGF-C have shown angiogenic activity. VEGFs signal through several membrane tyrosine kinase receptors which mediate their biological effects in vivo (Korpelainen and Alitalo 1998). Angiopoietin-1 and angiopoietin-2 are recently identified factors which may modify the response of VEGF gene therapy (Davis et al. 1996).

The family of fibroblast growth factors (FGF) can induce angiogenesis in vivo (Harada et al. 1994; Giordano et al. 1996). Most experience is with FGF-1, FGF-2 and FGF-5. FGF affects various types of cells in vivo, which differentiates it from VEGF, whose receptors are present mostly on endothelial cells and monocyte/macrophages (Korpelainen and Alitalo 1998; Ferrara and Buntling 1996). In addition to VEGFs and FGFs, several other factors, such as hepatocyte growth factor, have angiogenic activity which may bc utilized in clinical angiogenesis trials.

10.4 Clinical Trials

Human clinical trials with angiogenic proteins or gene therapy are listed in Table 1. It has recently been demonstrated that intravascular adenoviral gene transfer can lead to gene expression in human atherosclerotic arteries (Laitinen et al. 1998). Gene transfer efficiency with high titer adenovirus was 5%. Vascular smooth muscle cell was the main transfected cell type (Laitinen et al. 1998). Even though gene transfer efficiency was low, it demonstrated that gene transfer can be achieved in atherosclerotic human arteries in vivo.

First results from intramuscular $VEGF_{165}$ naked plasmid gene transfer in human peripheral vascular disease and severe angina pectoris have been described (Baumgartner et al. 1998; Losordo et al. 1998). Beneficial effects were reported with improvements in peripheral and myocardial blood flow and clinical condition of the patients. Recombinant FGF protein injection into the myocardium during bypass operations has also been reported to improve collateral formation in myocardium (Schumacher et al. 1998). Control hearts injected with inactivated FGF showed no growth of neovessels.

No serious adverse effects have been reported in any of these trials. Edema has been detected in legs treated with intramuscular VEGF gene therapy. Also, hypotension has been reported in some of these patients (Baumgartner et al. 1998).

Several therapeutic angiogenesis trials are currently underway (Table 1). These studies utilize both naked plasmids, plasmid/liposomes, and adenoviral vectors. Results from these early phase I and II gene therapy trials will significantly advance our understanding about the feasibility of angiogenic gene therapy in humans.

Acknowledgements. This work was supported by grants from the Finnish Foundation for Cardiovascular Research, the Kuopio University Hospital (EVO grants 5021, 5102, and 5130), and the Finnish Academy. The author also wishes to thank Ms Marja Poikolainen for preparing the manuscript.

Table 1. Angiogenic and restenosis gene therapy and recombinant protein trials

Investigator/ Company	Location	Started	Disease
Schumacher et al.	Klinik für Thorax-, Herz- und Gefässchirurgie, Fulda, Germany	1995	Coronary heart disease
Isner et al.	St. Elizabeth's Medical Center, Boston, USA	1994	Peripheral artery disease
Isner et al.	St. Elizabeth's Medical Center, Boston, USA	1995	Peripheral arterydisease, post PTA/DA restenosis
Isner et al.	St. Elizabeth's Medical Center, Boston, USA	1997	Coronary heart disease
Ylä-Herttuala et al.	Kuopio University Central Hospital, Kuopio, Finland	1996	Peripheral artery disease
Ylä-Herttuala et al.	Kuopio University Central Hospital, Kuopio, Finland	1998	Peripheral artery disease, post PTA restenosis
Ylä-Herttuala et al.	Kuopio University Central Hospital, Kuopio, Finland	1997	Coronary heart disease, post PTCA restenosis
Mann et al.	Multicenter trial, USA	1997	Vein graft stenosis,infrainguinal bypass operation
Crystal et al.	Cornell Medical Center, New York, USA	1997	Coronary heart disease, bypass operation
Simons et al.	Beth Israel Deaconess Medical Center, Boston, USA	1997	Coronary heart disease
Simons et al.	Beth Israel Deaconess Medical Center, Boston, USA	1997	Coronary heart disease, bypass operation
Collateral Therapeutics Inc	Multicenter trial, USA	1998	Coronary heart disease

PTA, percutaneous transluminal angioplasty; PTCA, percutaneous transluminal coronary angioplasty; DA, directional atherectomy
*Currently enrolling patients

Table 1. Angiogenic and restenosis gene therapy and recombinant protein trials

Delivery route	Treatment	Vector/ Protein	Patients (*n*)	Reference
Intramyocardial injection	bFGF	Recombinant protein	20	Schumacher et al. 1998
Intramuscular injection	VEGF	Naked DNA	9	Baumgartner et al. 1998
Hydrogel-coated balloon catheter after angioplasty	VEGF	Naked DNA	19	–
Intramyocardial injection	VEGF	Naked DNA	5	Losordo et al. 1998
Infusion-perfusion catheter after angioplasty	LacZ	Adenovirus	10	Laitinen et al. 1998
Infusion-perfusion catheter after angioplasty	VEGF	Plasmid-liposome/ adenovirus	25*	–
Infusion-perfusion catheter after angioplasty	LacZ/ VEGF	Plasmid-liposome/ adenovirus	40*	-
Direct pressurized soaking of the graft	E2F Decoy	Oligonucleotide	5	Mann et al. 1997 (abstract)
Intramyocardial injection	$VEGF_{121}$	Adenovirus	20*	–
Intracoronary injection	bFGF	Recombinant protein	52	–
Periarterial delivery with biodegradable matrix during bypass operation	bFGF	Recombinant protein	22	–
Intracoronary injection	FGF-4	Adenovirus	*	–

References

Baumgartner I, Pieczek A, Manor O, Blair R, Kearney M, Walsh K, Isner JM (1998) Constitutive expression of $VEGF_{165}$ after intramuscular gene transfer promotes collateral vessel development in patients with critical limb ischemia. Circulation 97:1114–1123

Davis S, Aldrich TH, Jones PF, Acheson A, Compton DL, Jain V, Ryan TE, Bruno J, Radziejewski C, Maisonpierre PC, Yancopoulos GD (1996) Isolation of angiopoietin-1, a ligand for the TIE2 receptor, by secretion-trap expression cloning. Cell 87:1161–1169

Ferrara N, Buntling S (1996) Vascular endothelial growth factor, a specific regulator of angiogenesis. Curr Opin Nephrol Hypertension 5:35–44

Giordano FJ, Ping P, McKirnan MD, Nozaki S, DeMaria AN, Dillmann WH, Mathieu-Costello O, Hammond HK (1996) Intracoronary gene transfer of fibroblast growth factor-5 increases blood flow and contractile function in an ischemic region of the heart. Nat Med 2:534–539

Harada K, Grossman W, Friedman M, Edelman ER, Prasad PV, Keighlcy CS, Manning WJ, Selke FW, Simons M (1994) Basic fibroblast growth factor improves myocardial function in chronically ischemic porcine hearts. J Clin Invest 94:623–630

Isner JM (1997) Angiogenesis and collateral formation. In: March KL (ed) Gene transfer in the cardiovascular system. Kluwer Academic, Boston, pp 307–330

Isner JM, Pieczek A, Schainfeld R, Blair R, Haley L, Asahara T, Rosenfield K, Razvi S, Walsh K, Symes JF (1996) Clinical evidence of angiogenesis after arterial gene transfer of $phVEGF_{165}$ in patient with ischemic limb. Lancet 348:370–374

Korpelainen EI, Alitalo K (1998) Signaling angiogenesis and lymphangiogenesis. Curr Opin Cell Biol 10:159–164

Laitinen M, Pakkanen T, Donetti E, Baetta R, Luoma J, Lehtolainen P, Viita H, Agrawal R, Miyanohara A, Friedmann T, Risau W, Martin JF, Soma M, Ylä-Herttuala S (1997) Gene transfer into the carotid artery using an adventitial collar: comparison of the effectiveness of the plasmid-liposome complexes, retroviruses, pseudotyped retroviruses, and adenoviruses. Hum Gene Ther 8:1645–1650

Laitinen M, Mäkinen K, Manninen H, Matsi P, Kossila M, Agrawal R, Pakkanen T, Luoma JS, Viita H, Hartikainen J, Alhava E, Laakso M, Ylä-Herttuala S (1998) Adenovirus-mediated gene transfer to lower limb artery of patients with chronic critical leg ischaemia. Hum Gene Ther 9:1481–1486

Losordo DW, Vale PR, Symes JF, Dunnington CH, Esakof DD, Maysky M, Ashare AB, Lathi K, Isner JM (1998) Gene therapy for myocardial angiogenesis. Initial clinical results with direct myocardial injection of phVEGF$_{165}$ as sole therapy for myocardial ischemia. Circulation 98:2800–2804

Mann MJ, Whittemore AD, Donaldson MC, Belkin MA, Orav EJ, Polak J, Dzau VJ (1997) Preliminary clinical experience with genetic engineering of human vein grafts: Evidence for target gene inhibition. (abstract) Circulation 96:I-4

Schumacher B, Pecher P, von Specht BU, Stegmann T (1998) Induction of neoangiogenesis in ischemic myocardium by human growth factors: first clinical results of a new treatment of coronary heart disease. Circulation 97:645–650

Ylä-Herttuala S (1997) Vascular gene transfer. Curr Opin Lipidol 8:72–76

Subject Index

Ernst Schering Research Foundation Workshop

Editors: Günter Stock
Ursula-F. Habenicht

Vol. 1 *(1991)*: Bioscience ⇋ Society – Workshop Report
Editors: D. J. Roy, B. E. Wynne, R. W. Old

Vol. 2 (1991): Round Table Discussion on Bioscience ⇋ Society
Editor: J. J. Cherfas

Vol. 3 (1991): Excitatory Amino Acids and Second Messenger Systems
Editors: V. I. Teichberg, L. Turski

Vol. 4 (1992): Spermatogenesis – Fertilization – Contraception
Editors: E. Nieschlag, U.-F. Habenicht

Vol. 5 (1992): Sex Steroids and the Cardiovascular System
Editors: P. Ramwell, G. Rubanyi, E. Schillinger

Vol. 6 (1993): Transgenic Animals as Model Systems for Human Diseases
Editors: E. F. Wagner, F. Theuring

Vol. 7 (1993): Basic Mechanisms Controlling Term and Preterm Birth
Editors: K. Chwalisz, R. E. Garfield

Vol. 8 (1994): Health Care 2010
Editors: C. Bezold, K. Knabner

Vol. 9 (1994): Sex Steroids and Bone
Editors: R. Ziegler, J. Pfeilschifter, M. Bräutigam

Vol. 10 (1994): Nongenotoxic Carcinogenesis
Editors: A. Cockburn, L. Smith

Vol. 11 (1994): Cell Culture in Pharmaceutical Research
Editors: N. E. Fusenig, H. Graf

Vol. 12 (1994): Interactions Between Adjuvants, Agrochemical and Target Organisms
Editors: P. J. Holloway, R. T. Rees, D. Stock

Vol. 13 (1994): Assessment of the Use of Single Cytochrome P450 Enzymes in Drug Research
Editors: M. R. Waterman, M. Hildebrand

Vol. 14 (1995): Apoptosis in Hormone-Dependent Cancers
Editors: M. Tenniswood, H. Michna

Vol. 15 (1995): Computer Aided Drug Design in Industrial Research
Editors: E. C. Herrmann, R. Franke

Vol. 16 (1995): Organ-Selective Actions of Steroid Hormones
Editors: D. T. Baird, G. Schütz, R. Krattenmacher

Vol. 17 (1996): Alzheimer's Disease
Editors: J.D. Turner, K. Beyreuther, F. Theuring

Vol. 18 (1997): The Endometrium as a Target for Contraception
Editors: H.M. Beier, M.J.K. Harper, K. Chwalisz

Vol. 19 (1997): EGF Receptor in Tumor Growth and Progression
Editors: R. B. Lichtner, R. N. Harkins

Vol. 20 (1997): Cellular Therapy
Editors: H. Wekerle, H. Graf, J.D. Turner

Vol. 21 (1997): Nitric Oxide, Cytochromes P 450,
and Sexual Steroid Hormones
Editors: J.R. Lancaster, J.F. Parkinson

Vol. 22 (1997): Impact of Molecular Biology
and New Technical Developments in Diagnostic Imaging
Editors: W. Semmler, M. Schwaiger

Vol. 23 (1998): Excitatory Amino Acids
Editors: P.H. Seeburg, I. Bresink, L. Turski

Vol. 24 (1998): Molecular Basis of Sex Hormone Receptor Function
Editors: H. Gronemeyer, U. Fuhrmann, K. Parczyk

Vol. 25 (1998): Novel Approaches to Treatment of Osteoporosis
Editors: R.G.G. Russell, T.M. Skerry, U. Kollenkirchen

Vol. 26 (1998): Recent Trends in Molecular Recognition
Editors: F. Diederich, H. Künzer

Vol. 27 (1998): Gene Therapy
Editors: R.E. Sobol, K.J. Scanlon, E. Nestaas, T. Strohmeyer

Vol. 28 (1999): Therapeutic Angiogenesis
Editors: J.A. Dormandy, W.P. Dole, G.M. Rubanyi

Supplement 1 (1994): Molecular and Cellular Endocrinology of the Testis
Editors: G. Verhoeven, U.-F. Habenicht

Supplement 2 (1997): Signal Transduction in Testicular Cells
Editors: V. Hansson, F. O. Levy, K. Taskén

Supplement 3 (1998): Testicular Function:
From Gene Expression to Genetic Manipulation
Editors: M. Stefanini et al.